MY WIFE HAS MULTIPLE SCLEROSIS

What Do I Do Now?

I0425966

Henry M. Rogers, III MBA

CreateSpace Edition

Table of Contents

ACKNOWLEDGEMENTS AND INTRODUCTION

My wife Martha was diagnosed on February 2004 with relapsing-remitting multiple sclerosis (RRMS). It was a real shocker, but nine years later, she is coping quite well with this disease. The fatigue, however, has progressed considerably. I started writing this book in 2006 and conducted countless hours of research to pull the MS facts together. I woke up at five in the morning and wrote for an hour each day. Over half of this book was written in about six months, but then life's events took precedence and my writing suffered from "not having enough time and focus." In June 2011, Martha and I decided we would relocate to Charleston, SC. That motivated me to finish this book and ensure its publishing. Martha possesses sheer determination and willpower to fight MS and I support her wholeheartedly.

This book is a testament to Martha's strong faith, determination, positive outlook, can-do attitude, and her inspiration to others out there suffering from this disabling disease. Multiple Sclerosis (MS) does not have to control your life or change your personality. You must learn how to adapt to the disease and still lead a rewarding life. Life with MS is frustrating, painful, depressing at times, challenging and unpredictable, but hope is out there if you look for it.

I encourage everyone who suffers from this unpredictable disease to *dig deep* and rely on your faith. For those husbands out there whose wives have MS, I hope this book provides you with some insight as to how you can better support your wife so that, together, you can combat this disease with a more positive and fulfilled approach to your lives. Your wife is depending upon you to support her in ways you never thought possible. Your life is also about to change considerably. I advise you to respond caringly and to avoid despair. Remember that *"when one door closes, another one opens."*

One must remember that God really never does give you more than you can handle. We just don't think we are ready to accept and face the challenges ahead until they are literally upon us. But when they happen, we discover that our minds and our ability to control our thoughts are the key. It is our determination and faith that will move mountains (you did not know you could move!) My grandfather used to say, *"The road to success is always under construction."* I love that saying. It rings so true.

I would like to thank all of my wife's health care providers who have proved exceptional through the tough times. These include Dr. Thomas Pellegrino, her first neurologist and friend from church (who died in Nov 2011), Dr. Patrick Parcells, her second neurologist, and his partners at Hampton Roads Neurology. Gratitude is also extended to Kim Meyers, Martha's infusion nurse at Hampton Roads Neurology. A final gratitude goes to Dr. Dawnielle Kerner, Martha's first ophthalmologist, who diagnosed Martha as most likely having MS after a flare-up of optic neuritis.

Martha has a new neurologist now since we moved to Mt. Pleasant, SC and his name is Dr. Ted Hughes with Tidewater Neurology. How fitting that is! Norfolk, or the

Hampton Roads area, was known as Tidewater, and here we are—seven hours and 463 miles away—and her new practice is named "Tidewater." And we knew a Dr. Ted Hughes in Norfolk, too!

We have wonderful drug companies today and we are blessed to have Biogen Idec. I would like to thank them for developing outstanding drugs like Avonex and Tysabri. Their Patient Advocate Program catapulted my wife to the forefront of MS Advocacy and provided her with the opportunity to tell her story to other MS patients in sponsored programs where she spoke with a physician. This 3rd edition includes the latest drug offerings to treat MS.

What can I say about families? Families are the first line of support. Both of our families rallied around us when Martha was diagnosed. Luckily, my parents and one of my sisters lived in our city, not too far from us. I know that they prayed for her diligently. I cannot say enough about the power of prayer. It works; try it! You will be pleased with the results! I thank my parents Henry and Carolyn Rogers for raising me up in the church so that I found my faith and learned to "give something back."

I also want to thank my sisters Amy Swink and Elaine Rogers-Hayes who both read the draft of this book at ninety-five percent completion and encouraged me to finish it. They felt it was a worthy effort and would motivate and inspire others facing similar circumstances. My gratitude also goes to my sisters-in-law, Jennifer Nice and Elizabeth (Liz) Smith, for also reading and critiquing this book.

I could not have completed this publication process without the aid of professional editing and book cover design. I would like to thank my editor, King Samuel Benson and graphic artists, Aubrey Watt, who designed my e-book cover and Hilary West, who designed my print book cover.

I would also like to thank Fr. Daniel Klem, our priest at Sacred Heart Catholic Church in Norfolk, who embraced Martha when she was newly diagnosed. He extended his support and the entire faith community at Sacred Heart showed their love and support to Martha during my extended work absence from home when she was newly diagnosed.

Special thanks go to our good friends at church whom we had coffee with after mass each week. I refer to them as the "coffee group." This group included Jane Pellegrino and her late husband Tom, Annette Field, Dean Reeder and his late wife Regina. Week after week, we shared life's stories and challenges, joked with each other and supported the collective endeavors of the group and each person. Each time, Martha and I felt inspired and consoled. We were a close-knit group and had dinner together often, told stories and enjoyed fine wine. As you may already know, life has a way of throwing many challenges your way. It is our response to these challenges that builds and defines one's character.

Finally, I want to thank my loving wife Martha who inspired me to write this book. Fifty percent of all profits from this book will be donated to the National Multiple Sclerosis Society specifically dedicated to research to end the devastating effects of this disease.

iv

Chapter 1

FACTS ABOUT MS YOU SHOULD KNOW

Multiple Sclerosis (MS) is an autoimmune disease that causes the body's central nervous system (CNS) to attack itself. MS is a disease in which the immune system mistakenly attacks the myelin coating of nerve fibers in the CNS, thus interfering with the brain's ability to send and receive messages. This destruction of myelin is called Demyelination. A common analogy of this condition is to think of the nerve fibers as electrical wires. Myelin is the insulated plastic coating on these wires. When it is "peeled" away, the electrical conduction of that wire is compromised, and can cause short circuiting. This is what happens with your nerves when MS destroys the myelin. The electrical impulses are disturbed. It is a chronic and progressive disease and sometimes disabling autoimmune disease. MS targets the brain, spinal cord and other components of the central nervous system.

Electrical impulses travel along nerve fibers called Axons. The axons connect the muscles and sensory fibers to the brain and spinal cord. Myelin is the protective sheath surrounding the axons. When the myelin is damaged, the signal is slowed down or interrupted when the electrical impulses travel to and from the brain and spinal cord. Multiple Sclerosis actually means "many scars," because scars or lesions in the brain and/or spinal cord occur when the myelin is damaged.

Multiple Sclerosis affects over 400,000 individuals in the United States and may affect as many as 2.5 million people world-wide. Every hour, in the US, another person is diagnosed with MS. MS mainly affects adults; however, approximately nine thousand children have also been diagnosed with MS. Approximately 70,000 individuals in the United Kingdom have MS. Approximately 50,000 people in Canada have MS. Scotland has the highest incidence per capita of MS in the world; 10,500 individuals have MS in Scotland. This equates to an incidence ratio of one in five hundred.

Twice as many women as men are diagnosed with this disease. Approximately seventy-five percent of the MS population is women. The specific reason for this is unknown; however, theories suggest it is due to hormonal reasons since the female body is designed to give birth. MS occurs more commonly in Caucasians, especially those of northern European ancestry.

Genetics does play a key role in MS. If one identical twin develops MS, the likelihood of the second twin developing MS is thirty percent. The incidence rate for non-identical twins, where one contracts multiple sclerosis, is approximately four percent. The risk of contracting MS if your father, mother or sibling has this disease is approximately three percent. If your father has the disease, your risk is approximately one percent, compared to two percent if your mother has the disease. Overall, the risk among the general population of contracting multiple sclerosis is approximately one in eight hundred.

MS was first described in 1868 by Jean-Martin Charcot. The real cause of MS is still unknown. No virus has ever been isolated as the cause of multiple sclerosis. Some theories suggest it may be an Epstein-Barr-like virus but this is unproven. Recent environmental studies indicate that MS may be caused by a persistent viral infection in the central nervous system or elsewhere in the body. It is theorized that there is some sort of "triggering" factor that is infectious and it must be encountered before the age of sixteen in order for the disease to be triggered in later life.

Also, where you live is important. If you have this infectious agent but move closer to the equator before the age of sixteen, your chances of developing MS in later life is significantly reduced. It is believed that some triggering factor in the environment causes MS to develop in people who are genetically predisposed to MS and live in northern temperate zones in North America and Europe.

Multiple sclerosis is five times more prevalent in temperate climates above the 37th parallel. Within the United States, a "dividing line" runs along the 37th parallel, from Newport News, Virginia, to Santa Cruz, California, along the northern border of North Carolina, the northern border of Arizona and across the top part of California. Below the 37th parallel, the incidence of Multiple Sclerosis is 57 to 78 cases per 100,000 people; above the 37th parallel, it is almost double. That equates to 110 - 140 cases per 100,000 people. Statistics have shown that if you have a genetic predisposition to contract the disease in one of these northern climates and then move south before the age of fifteen, your risk of developing MS is greatly reduced. After the age of fifteen, there is no difference if one relocates.

Ninety percent of MS patients are diagnosed between the ages of sixteen and sixty. The average age of onset is thirty to thirty-three years of age. Most people are thirty seven years old when diagnosed. Ten percent of those diagnosed are at least fifty years old. The average time between clinical onset of MS and diagnosis by physicians is between four and five years.

Multiple sclerosis affects everyone differently. Symptoms can vary widely across individuals for a number of reasons. When a clinical symptom presents, it can last a short or a long time, and may clear up completely. The reason for this is that the myelin that was damaged is able to heal itself. However, over time and with recurrent relapses, scars build up, and these lesions interfere with electrical impulses. Sometimes, the axon is damaged or severed, which results in permanent disability.

Three forms of multiple sclerosis exist; relapsing-remitting MS, secondary progressive MS, and primary progressive MS. Approximately eighty percent of people with MS have relapsing-remitting MS. This is characterized by flare-ups or relapses where one gradually recovers almost 100%. Over time, however, as more relapses occur, the recovery time is lengthened and the damage inflicted during the relapse contributes to long term disability since the body never fully recovers.

Secondary progressive MS behaves like relapsing-remitting MS in its early stages. It is characterized by frequent relapses and remissions, followed by noticeable physical and cognitive dysfunction. Relapses occur less frequently but the disability progresses. It is known that 50% of people who have relapsing-remitting MS will develop secondary progressive MS within ten years of initial diagnosis.

The third type of MS is primary progressive MS, which affects about 10% of the MS population. In this stage of MS, there are no relapses but physical and mental functions become progressively worse.

On average, thirty percent of women with multiple sclerosis have a relapse within three months of childbirth. During the early stages of the disease, complete or partial remission of symptoms will occur in about seventy percent of patients. Females tend to have more relapses than men.

Common symptoms of MS and its severity vary greatly since MS affects everyone differently. The most common problems include fatigue, poor vision, lack of co-ordination, weakness, speech and swallowing dysfunction, weakened bladder and bowel control, poor sexuality and cognitive function.

Fatigue and heat sensitivity are two of the most common and most troubling symptoms of MS. Fatigue occurs in about seventy-eight percent of MS patients. Sensory complaints such as tingling, swelling and numbness occur in up to fifty-five percent of MS patients and are the earliest signs and symptoms of MS in many cases. Blurry or double vision can occur. Unstable walking (ataxia) and dizziness (vertigo) occur in many individuals with MS. Weakness occurs in the legs often; therefore, physical therapy and strength training are recommended.   Approximately fifty percent of MS patients report extremity ataxia.

Spasticity occurs in the initial attack of MS in about forty-one percent of MS patients and is present in about sixty-two percent of patients with progressive MS. Bowel dysfunction occurs in approximately two-third of patients with MS. Cognitive and emotional dysfunctions occur in about fifty percent of MS patients.

Memory problems are also quite common and it is estimated that between two-third and three-fourth of MS patients suffer from varying forms of memory and reasoning problems. At least, seventy percent of women and ninety percent of men report some change in sexual function after the onset of the disease. Problems can range from decreased sexual drive to diminished orgasms, impaired sensations and decreased or loss of sexual drive.

Furthermore, the specific symptoms occurring are determined by the location of the lesion. Some lesions on the brain affect certain functions while lesions on the spinal cord affect other motor functions. Typical symptoms of balance, co-ordination and speech problems result from a lesion on the cerebrum and/or cerebellum. Muscle weakness, spasticity, paralysis, vision, bladder and bowel problems are due to lesions located along the motor nerve tracts. Sensory nerve tract lesions result in symptoms of altered sensation, numbness, prickling and burning sensations.

Only fifteen percent of patients present optic neuritis as a clinical symptom. About fifty percent of MS patients experience cognitive dysfunction. Constipation, bowel and bladder problems are common. Depression and

6

fatigue are the two most prevalent symptoms. Almost eighty percent of MS patients are heat sensitive and their symptoms will worsen if they become overheated. Once they cool down, however, they will immediately feel better.

Approximately seventy-five to eighty-five percent of patients with RRMS will eventually develop Secondary Progressive Multiple Sclerosis (SPMS). Roughly eighty percent of patients with MS experience fatigue. Approximately sixty percent of patients who have progressive disease will experience spasticity. Also, patients with MS have a greater risk of seizure than the general population. Approximately fifty-five percent of women will report some form of sexual dysfunction, compared to an average of eight-five percent for men.

At this time, there is no cure for multiple sclerosis; however, major strides have occurred over the past decade in both the understanding and diagnosis of the disease, and advancement in treatment options. Diagnosing MS became much easier with the introduction of Magnetic Resonance Imaging Technology (MRI) in 1973.

MRI is a non-invasive and usually painless diagnostic test where powerful magnetic field and radio waves are used to produce a computerized detailed image of the organs, soft tissues, bones and virtually all other internal organs and structures. Neurologists all agree that a thorough neurological exam coupled with an MRI has greatly aided their ability to diagnose MS. MRI results do not always reveal the severity of symptoms though. One person can have many lesions on the brain, black holes and Dawson's Fingers, but their symptoms can be mild.

On the other hand, a person can show significant mobility and cognitive impairment when the MRI shows only minor lesion activity.

Diagnosing MS involves both a clinical exam by a neurologist and confirmation by a diagnostic method (MRI, spinal tap, etc.) In the neurological exam, a detailed history is obtained and signs and symptoms are assessed. During the neurological exam, the physician will check for exaggerated reflexes and an eye examination will also be performed to determine any optic nerve damage. To diagnose a patient with MS, the neurologist must be able to find evidence of lesions in at least two distinct areas of the central nervous system, and must rule out any other illness similar to MS. This is where the MRI comes in today. It greatly aids in quickly ruling out or confirming MS following the neurological exam.

Studies have concluded that early intervention when one is newly diagnosed has a positive impact on long-term disability. Treating MS is two-fold; the first issue is to address the symptoms and to manage them; the second part of treatment is to change the progression and intensity of the disease by modifying the number and severity of attacks, and to minimize the progression of disability.

Tremendous advancement in the treatment of MS has occurred in recent years. In 1936, only about 8% of patients were reported to survive beyond twenty years of the onset of the illness. By 1961, over eighty percent of patients survived, at least twenty years, after the onset of the illness. By 2002, a patient diagnosed with multiple sclerosis can expect to live to average life expectancy minus seven years.

Significant progress has occurred in the last fifteen years in treating MS. The Food and Drug Administration (FDA) has approved six different drugs as disease-modifying agents since 1993. These include three drugs that are interferon-beta products; Betaserone, Avonex and Rebif. The other three drugs are Copaxone, Novantrone, and Tysabri.

Betaserone or 'interferon beta-1b', was the first drug of its type to be approved and marketed in the United States. It is marketed by Berlex Laboratories. The way it works is to shut down the inflammation of lesions in the brain. This drug has been proven to reduce relapse rate, decreases the intensity of the attacks, and reduces overall lesion activity. It is administered by subcutaneous injection (under the skin) every other day, and is the highest dose of interferon beta available. Betaserone is approved for relapsing-remitting MS.

Avonex has been proven to slow the progression of disability in relapsing-remitting MS patients. It also decreases the relapse rate. Avonex is administered weekly as an intramuscular injection at a lower dose than Betaserone or Rebif. Biogen Idec markets Avonex.

Rebif is identical to Avonex in structure; however it is administered in higher and more frequent doses as a subcutaneous injection. Rebif has been proven to reduce the number and severity of relapses, delays progression of disability and also reduces the number of new and overall lesions. Canada and Europe have been using Rebif and it has only recently been approved by the FDA for marketing in the US. Rebif is marketed by Serono, Inc.

Copaxone is different from beta interferon in structure and performance. It is a glatiramer acetate product. Copaxone is basically a group of amino acids that resemble myelin. It suppresses the immune system from attacking itself. It decreases the frequency and severity of attacks, similar to Betaserone and Rebif, but is less effective on existing lesions. It also is a subcutaneous injection and is administered daily. It is marketed by Teva Neuroscience.

Tysabri, or 'Natalizumab', is a human monoclonal antibody. Tysabri actually blocks the receptor on the white blood cell which aids its attraction to the blood-brain barrier. Therefore, Tysabri acts to decrease inflammation in the brain by preventing inflammatory activity from occurring. It is administered by IV infusion once every four weeks. Tysabri has been proven to slow the progression of disability and the relapse rate is reduced by two-third. Thus, it is the most effective drug available to combat MS. It is recommended for patients who cannot tolerate or have not responded well to the other disease-modifying drugs. Tysabri is marketed by Biogen Idec and Elan Pharmaceuticals.

Novantrone, or 'mitoxantrone', is a chemotherapy drug that slows the progression of MS and reduces relapses. It suppresses the activity of T and B cells. These are white blood cells that attack the myelin. Novantrone is prescribed for patients with secondary progressive MS or worsening relapsing remitting MS. It is administered by IV infusion once every three months for a period of two years. A cardiac evaluation is usually performed prior to beginning treatment, as it does affect the heart. Novantrone is marketed by Immunex Corporation.

During an acute relapse, steroids can be used to shorten the duration of the exacerbation. Steroids do not affect the relapse rate but do reduce the inflammation quickly. Steroids can be administered by IV infusion for a period of three to five days typically. Oral doses can also be prescribed. These steroids include prednisone, prednisolone, methylprednisolone, betamethason, and dexamethasone.

Since 1998, the treatment of MS has changed significantly, due primarily to the advancement in platform drug therapy. Quality of life can be improved in MS patients. Early intervention appears to be the key. Once you are diagnosed with MS, begin treatment immediately with one of the available drugs. This early treatment can have a profound impact on long term disability.

One of the most noticeable symptoms in MS patients is their gait. Many MS patients need a wider gait to maintain their balance. Walking stability and speed are also apparent in that MS patients often times walk slower than normal.

Ampyra (dalfampridine) is used for improving walking in patients with MS. Ampyra was approved by the FDA for MS treatment in January 2010. Benefits of Ampyra in MS is demonstrated by an increase in walking speed. Although its mechanism of action in MS is not fully understood, Ampyra is a potassium channel blocker.

In animal studies, Ampyra improved conduction of impulses in damaged nerves by blocking potassium channels. In clinical trials Ampyra improved walking speed more than placebo. In one clinical study, 34.8% of Ampyra treated patients experienced improved walking as compared with 8.3% of placebo recipients. In a separate study, 42.9% of Ampyra recipients showed improved walking speed versus 9.3% for the placebo group.

Ampyra is administered orally twice daily without regard to food. Ampyra is available in 10 mg tablets which must be swallowed whole. Patients with a history of seizures, or moderate or severe renal failure should not use Ampyra.

Common side effects of Ampyra include urinary tract infection, insomnia (difficulty sleeping), dizziness, headache, nausea, constipation, back pain, balance disorder, MS relapse, nasopharyngitis, heartburn, weakness, throat pain and burning, and tingling or itchiness of skin. Ampyra has not been adequately evaluated in pregnancy and is classified as FDA pregnancy risk category C. Due to the lack of conclusive safety data, Ampyra should only be used during pregnancy if the potential benefit justifies the potential harm to the fetus.

Just in the last several years, new infusion, injectable, and oral drugs have been approved by the FDA. The new oral drugs that have been approved by the FDA in recent years include: Gilenya (fingolimod), Aubagio (teriflunomide), and Tecfidera (dimethyl fumarate or DMF). Gilenya is the first oral medication approved for the treatment of relapsing-remitting MS. Gilenya was approved by the FDA in September 2010.

Gilenya helps to decrease the frequency of acute attacks and delays the accumulation of physical disability. Gilenya is a sphingosine 1-phosphate receptor modulator and is thought to help reduce the number of lymphocytes (white blood cells) in the peripheral blood. Although the exact mechanism by which Gilenya helps to treat MS is unknown, it may be related to its involvement in reducing the migration of white blood cells into the brain and spinal cord. The effectiveness of treatment with Gilenya was demonstrated in the TRANSFORMS trial that compared oral Gilenya (0.5 mg orally once a day) to intramuscular interferon beta-1a (30 mcg once weekly) for a period of 12 months. The annualized relapse rate was significantly lower in the Gilenya recipients at 0.16 versus 0.33 for the interferon beta-1a recipients.

The usual recommended dose of Gilenya is 0.5 mg orally once a day without regard to food. Initiation of treatment with Gilenya may cause a decrease in the heart rate. Therefore, the first dose of Gilenya must be administered in a clinical setting where the patient is observed by healthcare providers for at least 6 hours.

The most common side effects of treatment include headache, influenza, diarrhea, back pain, an increase in liver enzymes and cough. Other significant side effects which have been reported in clinical trials and require monitoring include: a drop in white blood cell counts, macular retinal edema (eye problems), AV block (abnormal conduction in the heart), and the risk for infections. Also, when given with oral ketoconazole (an azole antifungal), there is a concern for increased blood levels of Gilenya and the consequent risk for side effects. Because Gilenya may reduce the immune response to vaccines, administration of live attenuated vaccines should be avoided during and for 2 months after stopping treatment with Gilenya. Use of Gilenya during pregnancy should be avoided if possible due to concerns for causing harm to the fetus. Additionally, women of child bearing potential are advised to use effective contraceptive methods during and for at least 2 months after stopping Gilenya.

On September 12, 2012, the FDA approved a new multiple sclerosis treatment called Aubagio (teriflunomide), a once-a-day tablet for the treatment of adults with relapsing forms of multiple sclerosis (MS).

"In a clinical trial, the relapse rate of patients using Aubagio was about 30 percent lower than the rate for those taking a placebo," said Russell Katz, M.D., director of the Division of Neurology Products in the FDA's Center for Drug Evaluation and Research. "Multiple sclerosis can impair movement, sensation, and thinking, so it is important to have a variety of treatment options available to patients."

The most common side-effects of Aubagio experienced by patients in clinical trials include diarrhea, abnormal liver tests, nausea, and hair loss. The drug contains a Boxed Warning to alert prescribers and patients to the risk of liver problems, including death, and a risk of birth defects. Physicians should do blood tests to check liver function before a patient starts taking Aubagio and also periodically during treatment. Also included in the Boxed Warning is an alert noting that, based on animal studies, the drug may cause fetal harm. For this reason, Aubagio is labeled as Pregnancy Category X, which means women of childbearing age must have a negative pregnancy test before starting the drug and use effective birth control during treatment. Aubagio will be dispensed with a patient Medication Guide that provides important instructions on its use and drug safety information. Aubagio is made by Bridgewater, N.J.-based Sanofi Aventis.

Tecfidera is an oral medication used to treat relapsing forms of MS, and was approved by the FDA in March 2013. The exact mechanism by which Tecfidera provides therapeutic benefits in MS is not known but is appears to have neuroprotective and anti-inflammatory properties. Evidence of clinical effectiveness of Tecfidera treatment was provided in the "Efficacy and Safety Study of Oral Tecfidera (BG-12) with Active Reference in Relapsing Remitting Multiple Sclerosis (CONFIRM)" study that showed that Tecfidera decreased the annualized relapse rate by 44% at twice daily dosing and 51% at three times daily dosing. Similarly, in the "Determination of the Efficacy and Safety of Oral BG-12 in Relapsing-Remitting MS" study, Tecfidera decreased the annualized relapse rate by 47% with 240 mg twice daily dosing and 52% with 240 mg three times daily dosing.

Treatment with Tecfidera is usually started with 120 mg orally twice a day for 7 days followed by 240 mg twice daily thereafter. Tecfidera is available in 120 mg and 240 mg delayed release capsules which should not be crushed, chewed, or broken. Capsules may be taken with or without food; however taking with food may decrease the incidence of flushing. The most common side effects of treatment are flushing, stomach pain, diarrhea, and nausea. These side effects usually decrease over the first month of treatment. Other reported side effects include itching, a drop in white blood cell counts, increase in liver enzymes, and loss of protein in the urine. Due to the potential risk of causing harm to the fetus, Tecfidera should be avoided in pregnancy if possible.

Plegridy (Plegridy), is the newest formulation of interferon beta-1a drugs, and was approved by the FDA in August 2014. As Plegridy requires fewer injections, it may be better tolerated than the nonpeglyated interferon formulations. The exact mechanism by which Plegridy exerts its therapeutic benefits in MS is unknown but is thought to be similar to that of the other interferons. As such, peginterferon is thought to decrease inflammation and have neuroprotective effects.

Approval of Plegridy was based on the results of the ADVANCE clinical trial which compared peginterferon (125 mcg every 2 weeks or every 4 weeks) to placebo. The annualized relapse rate at 48 weeks was 0.256 for the peginterferon every 2 week group, 0.288 for the every 4 week group, and 0.397 for the placebo group. Additionally, peginterferon treatment was associated with statistically significant improvements in reducing disability progression and brain lesions.

Plegridy is administered subcutaneously every 14 days. The recommended dose is 125 mcg every 14 days, with most patients titrated as follows; 63 mcg on day 1, then 94 mcg on day 15, and finally 125 mcg (full dose) on day 29. The most common side effects of treatment are injection site reactions (pain, redness, or itching), flu-like symptoms, fever, headache, muscle pain, chills, joint pain, and weakness. Other reported side effects include liver disease, depression, seizures, allergic or anaphylactic reactions, decrease in blood counts, and worsening of heart disease. Plegridy is not recommended for use during pregnancy due to the potential risk of causing harm to the fetus.

Lemtrada (alemtuzumab) is administered by intravenous infusion, and was approved by the FDA in November 2014. Lemtrada is a humanized monoclonal antibody directed against the CD52 antigen. The CD52 antigen is found on the surface of numerous cells in the body including white blood cells, NK cells, monocytes, macrophages, platelets, and others.

Lemtrada is used to treat relapsing forms of MS and is generally reserved for patients who have failed to adequately respond to two or more MS treatments. In the CARE-MS clinical trial, Lemtrada proved to be more effective than interferon beta-1a in reducing the relapse rate in patients with relapsing-remitting MS (RRMS). The annualized relapse rate was 0.18 for the Lemtrada group versus 0.39 for the interferon beta-1a group. Similar findings were also demonstrated in the CARE-MS II study which evaluated adult patients with RRMS who had experienced at least one relapse while being treated with interferon beta-1a or glatiramer. At 2 years, Lemtrada was superior in reducing relapse and the progression of disability.

Lemtrada is administered by intravenous infusion at 12 mg/day over 4 hours for two treatment courses. The first treatment course is given once daily for 5 consecutive days (60 mg total dose), followed by the second treatment course 12 months later for 3 consecutive days (36 mg total dose). Due to the significant risk of infusion reactions (infusion reactions occurred in approximately 90% of patients), patients are premedicated with high dose corticosteroids (1000 mg of methylprednisolone or equivalent) immediately prior to infusion and for the first 3 days of each treatment course. Additionally, patients must also receive prophylaxis for herpes and pneumocystis jirovecii pneumonia (PCP) during treatment and for several weeks after.

HIV-infected patients should not use Lemtrada. The most common side effects of Lemtrada treatment are rash, headache, fever, nausea, common cold, urinary tract infection, fatigue, insomnia, upper respiratory tract infection, herpes viral infection, hives, itching, thyroid gland disorders, fungal infection, arthralgia (joint pain), pain in the extremity, back pain, diarrhea, sinusitis, mouth pain or sore throat, paresthesia (tingling, pricking, burning sensations in the skin), dizziness, stomach pain, flushing and vomiting. Due to the potential risk of causing harm to the fetus, Lemtrada should be avoided in pregnancy if possible. Lemtrada was approved by the FDA in November 2014 for the treatment of RRMS. In addition to treating MS, Lemtrada is also used to treat chronic lymphocytic leukemia (CLL), a type of blood cancer.

Chapter 2

THE INITIAL DIAGNOSIS

For some people, a conclusive diagnosis of multiple sclerosis can take months or even years. Martha was diagnosed as having MS fairly quickly. She had an acute attack of optic neuritis in late January 2004. At the time, she was working as a substitute teacher for Norfolk Collegiate School and was also a special projects manager. I remember her coming home each day totally exhausted and agitated. She stated that she felt like she had headache that may be due to a sinus infection. Her vision was getting blurry, especially in the left eye. Additionally, Martha was unsteady on her feet. Just going to work was now a challenge for her. Increasingly, my concerns mounted about her situation.

Martha made an appointment with her primary care physician, Dr. Thomas Joyce, at Little Creek Medical Associates. He diagnosed her as having a sinus infection and prescribed some antibiotics. So Martha took them and continued working. She did not feel any better a week to ten days later. The antibiotics should have taken their course by then.

Her colleagues at work started to notice a significant change in her gait; she was dragging her left foot. She did not have a desk of her own so she had to carry her books and papers in her "mobile office," which was a small briefcase on wheels. One of the wheels, however, had become cracked and it was not rolling well. So she had to pull it a bit down the hall. Martha did not make me aware of this until a few weeks later. I was able to repair the wheel.

Martha likewise started dropping papers and books frequently. Her left eye continued to worsen, until her vision was cloudy and extremely blurry. Folks at work told her she should see an ophthalmologist. When she told me this at home that day, I pulled out the yellow pages. I remembered that an ophthalmologist had an office at Depaul Medical Center, right across the street from our house. Martha was able to book an appointment quickly with Dr. Dawnielle Kerner.

At the time, I was working as a contractor at Ft. Eustis. Life was stressful then as our van had been stolen and we were down to one vehicle. My parents were out of town and we were able to borrow their car.

On the day of Martha's appointment, she decided not to risk driving my mother's car since her eyes would be dilated so she walked across Granby Street to the office since it was close and the weather was not too cold. Dr. Kerner performed an extensive eye exam and seemed concerned. The doctor ordered a brain MRI to conclude her diagnosis. She thought Martha could have a brain tumor. And Martha, being the type of person she is, asked the doctor her initial prognosis, which was not good.

So with her eyes dilated and the "big ole" sunglasses you receive to wear to protect your eyes from the sun, Martha left the doctor's office and walked home. As she recalls, it was a tenuous walk home, with her eyes dilated and feeling unsteady on her feet. Martha hoped and prayed that she did not trip and fall down and get mowed down in the middle of Granby Street while crossing it on the way home. Cars travel close to fifty miles an hour on Granby Street even though the speed limit is thirty five miles per hour. When she arrived home, Elizabeth, our oldest daughter who was seventeen, had one of her friends over and they laughed at Martha with the sunglasses on.

When I returned home from work that day, Martha and I engaged in a serious discussion about the current situation. Our youngest daughter Sarah, fifteen, overheard us talking in the kitchen. The only words that stuck in her mind were "brain tumor." Martha was explicit with Sarah. She reminded her, "Sarah, we do not know for sure, but the doctor thinks Mommy may have a brain tumor. The MRI will confirm or deny this in a few days. Do not tell anybody at school."

I lay in bed that night, thinking about what I had told Martha a week earlier when she complained about her headaches. I had jokingly said, "Honey, maybe you have a brain tumor."

I now regretted those remarks since she actually may have a tumor. We prayed briefly and remained calm but concerned. We would just have to wait for the MRI results.

While we were waiting to have the MRI performed, Martha continued to work. The next day when she went to school, people were remarking, "Martha, we are so sorry you may have a brain tumor."

A gift basket also arrived from a collegiate parent when she returned home from work that day. Obviously, our words of warning to Sarah not to tell anyone were not heeded at all!

The MRI was performed several days later at Depaul Medical Center. Martha mentioned this to Dr. Pellegrino at church that Sunday, and he said he would be able to get a copy of the impression on Monday and he would call us and let us know the results. He did not call us, however. Martha was anxious as to why he did not call. Dr. Kerner called on Monday and asked us to come to the office on Tuesday and wanted us to meet with her.

I remember rushing home from Ft. Eustis, fighting the traffic in order to arrive by 3 o'clock for her appointment. Martha recalls that when she was in the waiting room by herself, she could hear the front desk clerks talking about her. Apparently, her case was rather high profile since they initially thought she had a brain tumor. The doctor called Martha back into the examination room. I called her on the cell phone while I was pulling into the parking lot and she told me that she was meeting with Dr. Kerner. I rushed into the office a few minutes later.

I was present when Dr. Kerner came in and remarked to my wife, "Well, I never thought I would be so happy to tell one of my patients they most likely had MS, but in your case, that is a better option because I really was worried that you had a brain tumor."

She stated that Dr. Pellegrino would meet with us tomorrow and perform his initial exam on Martha and then discuss treatment options. Dr. Kerner did not discuss MS in detail; only to say that treatment options were much better today and that Martha was lucky to have Dr. Pellegrino as her neurologist.

Dr. Pellegrino was a practicing neurologist at the largest neurology practice in Norfolk. He was well-respected; an outstanding general neurologist with quite a number of MS patients. He did not profess to be an expert on MS but he was very experienced and knowledgeable in the treatment of MS patients. His practice did not have an MS expert on staff at the time.

We met with Dr. Pellegrino the next day and he performed his initial exam on her and concluded that she had probably had MS for a few years before it presented itself with the clinical attack of optic neuritis. During the exam, a detailed history is necessary and Martha told Dr. Pellegrino that her first cousin had MS. Thus, she had a genetic predisposition to the disease. She was born in Newport News and lived in Richmond and Lynchburg, so she had always lived in Virginia.

According to a 2004 census, the population of Virginia was approximately 7,459,827. The estimated total number of people with disabilities in Virginia was 1,491,965. This equates to a total disability ratio of one in five. And of those disabled, 8,877 have Multiple Sclerosis. This equates to a .06 percent incidence of MS to total disabilities statewide, which is not that large. Martha, however, was now one of those 8,877 individuals in Virginia with MS. Life would no longer be the same.

During Martha's initial neurological exam, treatment options were discussed. Dr. Pellegrino recommended one of the platform drugs (Avonex, Rebif, and Copaxone) but he let us make the decision which drug to use. The most important treatment decision, he explained, was "to begin drug therapy immediately."

"All of these drugs do basically the same thing," he said, "but Copaxone is a bit different in how it works."

He told us that Avonex was a weekly injection. Once we heard weekly versus daily injections as a treatment option, our minds were made up. He gave us a patient kit to take home and review so we could make our final decision. We decided there that we were leaning towards Avonex, so he gave us that kit.

Martha ordered Avonex the very next day. A visit was scheduled with the nurse who came to our house to instruct us on how to administer the injection. The nurse demonstrated how to inject the drug into the muscle. She suggested the thigh muscle. We planned for me to inject Martha. My oldest daughter Elizabeth was also present for the patient education session. Since she wanted to become a physician assistant or nurse practitioner one day, we felt it would be beneficial to her so she'd be able to inject her mother in my absence. The most difficult part of the whole process, in my opinion, was taking the cap of the needle off. I have stubby fingers and often chewed my nails, so it was tough for me to do this. After several attempts, I succeeded in taking the cap off.

Martha took the first couple of doses in her legs. She would alternate legs each week. But she complained of muscle aches and pains in her legs and found it painful to walk the next day. So, after two injections, we decided to switch to the muscle in her arm, on the outside of the bicep region. This worked much better for her.

Within a month of Martha being diagnosed with MS, I was called out of town by my job for a period of three months. I came home just one weekend in every two weeks. Martha and Elizabeth decided it was too upsetting and difficult to do the injections at home. Martha did not want to inject herself, so she decided she would take the drugs to Dr. Pellegrino's office and the nurse would administer the weekly dose of Avonex. This approach worked well for us during those stress-filled periods when I was not home to give her the injections.

While I was away, Martha called me around five o'clock in the morning without fail, to rehash the events of the previous day and her anxiety about what was in store for her that day. She was still working full-time. And since Sarah 'spilled the beans', Martha had to tell her boss, Will King, the headmaster of Norfolk Collegiate School that she did not have a brain tumor, but that she had MS. I remember Martha telling me that she told him, "Will, I have good news and bad news. The good news is that I don't have a brain tumor."

Will then responded, "Thank God!"

Martha continued, "The bad news is that I have multiple sclerosis."

He said, "Oh my God. I am sorry to hear that, but I am relieved it is not a brain tumor."

Telling your employer that you have MS is a sticky situation. Labor law attorneys will advise you not to tell them right away, but in Martha's case she had no choice. Over time, she would be able to receive accommodations. Martha was very fortunate. Not all employers are as kind as Norfolk Collegiate was to Martha.

I felt strange and powerless knowing that I was not at home where she needed me. My two teenage daughters were trying to adjust to life at home without me. It was extremely stressful and upsetting. Both kids would not really discuss the situation with Martha or me. We deduced that the kids were both perplexed and a bit scared about the whole situation and did not know how to act. All I could do was to pray for my family during the day and then talk with each of them at night.

The faith community at Sacred Heart Church in Norfolk provided my wife with tremendous loving support especially during the first six months after being newly diagnosed. The most important action I took was to pray since I was out of town a lot during those first three months.

Father Dan and the parish community embraced and prayed for Martha during this turning point in her life. 2004 was a special year for us, especially during Lent. Martha was asked to carry the "oil of the sick" at the procession of the oils on Holy Thursday at Mass.

Martha's close network of friends were shocked to learn of her diagnosis but quickly responded. Surprisingly, not too many of my friends called me to find out how I was doing with this whole situation. That is understandable; however, the caregiver has a significant role to play in aiding his wife in coping with this disease. It is not easy for us caregivers, either. We get scared at times and ponder what could or may happen down the road. Personally, I do not think about this much. My attitude is, "I will confront those challenges if and when they may occur in the future." Life is challenging enough coping with the issues of today, so I do not waste time or energy on things that are out of my control. You cannot control what happens to you in life; all you CAN control is your response to situations and the people around you.

Many of my conversations with Martha in the first few months were focused on the "Why did I have to come down with MS?" I relied on God to help us weather the storm. Often, I would have to redirect Martha's thoughts to "How are we going to get through this," rather than "Why did this happen to me?" I would have to say, in retrospect, that this is going to be your wife's first significant hurdle to overcome with a diagnosis of multiple sclerosis.

Chapter 3

BALL DOG BELLE

Many people say things happen for a reason and life is not just about coincidence and circumstance. I believe that our lives are the product of our choices—good and bad. There is a consequence to every action and this seems logical to me; it is how the universe is ordered—by natural laws. Usually, God reveals his redemptive self when, as the saying goes, "bad things happen to good people."

Many years ago, I actually read this book titled <u>When Bad Things Happen to Good People</u>. It is an excellent book and I highly recommend it to anyone who's in a terrible situation they know they don't deserve. My point is this: Martha's father, Bernie, died of prostate cancer in 1999, but during the last six months of his life, he decided to buy his wife Charlotte a dog that would bring her joy and comfort her while serving as her "therapy dog." Through this process, we also got a dog (Charlotte's dog's sister). Our dog was named Belle. Martha and I often reflect on how our dog Belle truly was a "gift from God."

Bernie was astute and planned ahead. He knew that Charlotte would love that dog more than any other dog in the world. That dog would be so special because of its significance. As I mentioned, Martha is from Lynchburg. When Bernie decided to get Charlotte a dog, they both agreed on the breed; an English springer spaniel. They had researched this breed and fell in love with this type of dog for several reasons. First, the spaniel has a calm disposition and is a great family dog. Secondly, the spaniel loves exercise and Charlotte loved to walk. Thirdly, the spaniel has such soulful and kind eyes. And finally, they are just so darn cute, especially as puppies.

Martha went to the breeding grounds in Bedford County with her sister Becky to pick out a dog for Charlotte. When she arrived, she found eight of the cutest little Springer pups you have ever laid eyes on. There was one dog in particular that kept running up to Martha. She would hold her and then put her down and go towards another pup and this one pup just kept coming back. In Martha's words, this dog "chose her."

When she told the story to Bernie, he said, "You have to have that dog. Go back tomorrow and pick out another dog for your mother. I will buy that puppy for you. Let's call Hank and test the waters to see if he is amenable to getting a dog right now. I don't want to upset him if he is not ready for you to have a dog right now."

Martha called me and told me the story and all I recall saying in my state of shock was; "Absolutely not! It is not the right time for a dog. I appreciate the offer, but getting a dog is like raising a kid. It is a lot of responsibility and we have too much going on right now to add a puppy to the mix."

I told Martha I did not think we were ready for a dog then, because I knew I would be the one to train it. I had a dog when I was a kid; it was a German short-haired Pointer named Champ. He was a great bird dog, so I was very comfortable training it. But I and Martha's life situation just did not fit well with introducing a puppy into the mix at that time. Martha kept pressing me until I finally retorted, "Absolutely not! I forbid it!"

But once Martha emphatically spelt it out to me that WE WERE GETTING A DOG, I accepted it. My focus was then on choosing the proper name. You need to understand something about Martha; once she makes up her mind to do something, there is no stopping her regardless of whatever you tell her. Fifteen years of marriage then had taught me that. Learn to pick your battles!

The name I decided on was "Belle" which stands for Bernie Ever Lasting Love Eternal. Belle was a special pup indeed. I never thought I could love a dog so much. Everything serves a particular purpose and having this dog as a gift from Bernie brought our family immense joy and love, and his memory will continue to warm our hearts.

Well, to this day, we both laugh at how silly I had been in saying the "absolutely not" comment. I "absolutely" and unequivocally loved that dog. I embraced Belle and trained her to be very obedient. She was a wonderful dog. I gave her a tennis ball in the yard and she amused herself for hours, playing with it. She would dexterously use her paws to shuffle the ball around and push it through the gate where it adjoined the fence. Then she would proceed to "stare it down" and start barking at it until you threw it back into the fenced off yard for her. This routine was repeated relentlessly. I honestly believe that when she was sleeping, which was most of the time, she was dreaming. Belle would let out the cutest little yelps and her paws would flinch and her cute little mouth would twitch. That is when you knew that she was dreaming about playing with a tennis ball.

When Martha was diagnosed and I was out of town, Belle took care of Martha. She would get up in the bed with her in my spot and keep her company. Martha said, for the first few weeks after I was gone, that Belle would pine at the front door, waiting for her master to arrive, but to no avail.

We called Belle an "angel with fur." She truly was a love machine. She was stunningly beautiful and then had such personality to accompany her good looks. She was the full canine package!

The calming effect that Belle projected to Martha was tremendous. Being newly diagnosed with Multiple Sclerosis is scary and not having your spouse with you complicated matters. Physicians have proven that stress is actually physically harmful to the body; stress triggers even more harmful reactions in your body when you have MS since your immune system is already working double time.

Petting a dog and having a dog as a companion is therapeutic. This is why therapy dogs visit nursing homes and hospitals. They have been proven to provide a calming and temporary healing effect on the residents, reducing their stress and filling their hearts with love and joy.

Belle followed Martha around the house at all times. She was there by her side, whatever she did. When Martha lay in bed, Belle climbed into the bed with her. Just hearing her snore at night and all her many cute sounds helped Martha feel more settled. We remarked often how we just loved to hear all of Belle's sounds at night when she slept in our room.

The adjustment process one undergoes when newly diagnosed with MS is significant. Martha was grappling with a myriad of emotional and physical changes; finding the proper balance for antidepressant medications and anti-fatigue medications, experiencing the sexual side effects of these drugs, and battling frequent bouts of anger and depression, to name a few. Her phone calls to me in the early mornings were pensive but a bit calmer as we would talk about her day before and how much she missed me, but that she was overjoyed to have Belle up in the bed with her.

Martha remarked on numerous occasions, "I don't know how I could have made it through that period when you were gone if I did not have Belle to keep me company. She took care of me. She knew I was sick. She is an angel with fur."

I think that sums up how we felt about Belle. Her personality was effervescent and she was the cutest thing when she played with the tennis ball. We enjoyed walking her, and walking greatly improved Martha's physical strength and ability to cope with MS. As I have mentioned, to fight this disease requires both physical and mental fortitude.

Chapter 4

PREPARING YOURSELF MENTALLY

The Kubler-Ross grief cycle applies to adjusting to life with MS once your wife has been diagnosed with MS. Dr. Elisabeth Kubler-Ross explains in her theory that there are five stages of grief that individuals must experience during painful periods in their life. This can include the loss of a loved one or the loss of something dear to that person. These stages are: denial and isolation, anger, bargaining, depression and finally, acceptance.

During the denial and isolation phase, an individual tends to deny that the loss has occurred. Withdrawal from social contacts is common.

Upon being diagnosed with MS, your wife is "losing her normal life." Studies have shown that many women who have MS are driver-type personalities. They are used to being strong and productive members of society and contributors in their families. So, for them to accept this life-changing disease is difficult, to say the least. It was understandable, then, for her to deny losing this normal self.

For the first few months, Martha would constantly ponder: "Why did I have to get MS? Haven't I been through enough in my life already? I broke my neck in 1994, lost my father in 1999 and suffered through your failed business venture in 2002."

Martha's denial phase was one of shock and disbelief initially. "How could this happen to me," she would remark. "I just cannot understand why this had to happen to me? I am too old to get MS."

It was very disconcerting that my wife was poised to endure yet more significant challenges. All I could say to her was, "Honey, we can do this. You can do this. It is not like you have cancer. MS is treatable and you will not die with MS. I will help you get through this."

Those words did not do much good, however. She had to accept them in her mind first. She was not ready to accept it yet. This is normal.

In Martha's case, the denial quickly turned to anger. She reflected on the major events in her life over the last several years, now understanding why she felt so terrible in the heat and why she was so fatigued every day after work. It became clear to both of us that she had had MS for quite some time without ever presenting with a clear clinical attack. We concluded that she had the initial onset of MS with extreme fatigue about two years prior to her official diagnosis in February 2004. The more she reflected on how hard she had been working for the last two years (with MS but did not know it at the time), the angrier she became.

Working full time during those two years was draining her energy. She would come home totally exhausted. So, in her case, fatigue was affecting her greatly.

I did not understand what was happening. All I knew was that my wife was not very happy working. We needed the money and so she continued working, but it was taking a toll on her physically and emotionally. Martha was just like her father, Bernie. I teased her often, calling her "Bernadette." Bernie was "go, go, go, all the time." He never stopped until he fell asleep, exhausted after the day's activities.

This pace continued for about two years. Summertime was especially challenging for us since we did not understand yet why Martha felt so bad when she was outside in the heat. We used to have a little eighteen foot center console boat. Martha loved to go cruising but once we got out on the water, in the heat of the day, she would start to feel sick to her stomach. We adjusted the schedule to earlier in the morning or late in the afternoon when there was a breeze and it was not too hot. We used to go to Willoughby Beach frequently. I would launch the boat at the 15th Street ramp, drive the boat around the bridge tunnel, and then anchor up close to the beach and swim in. We would sit on the beach for a while and then take a boat ride. I would take the kids tubing also. They enjoyed that greatly.

I will never forget the one day back in 2003 when I was at this spot in Willoughby and had the boat anchored in the water about fifty yards off the beach. Over the next hour or so, I noticed that the boat looked like it was getting lower in the water. It did not look good, so I quickly swam out there and started the boat up. Little did I know that the external plug was missing! I jammed the throttle forward. The boat was so heavy-laden with water that it took a while to plane, despite the engine being a Yamaha 150 HP.

When a boat has that much water in the bilge, it does not get up "out of the hole" very quickly. I finally managed to drain all the water out of the boat and quickly drove to the ramp to pull it up. Once on the trailer, I witnessed water 'gushing' out the transom where the plug was missing. Mystery solved.

I was trying to sell the boat that earlier year and had it on consignment at Budget Boats. I never took out the external plug, always leaving it in. When the boat did not sell, I picked it up and launched it for a test ride as usual. I thought it may have a new leak that might have occurred when the boat dealer launched the boat. The bilge pump always seemed to run when I was not moving. Little did I know that someone had stolen the external plug when it was on consignment at Budget Boats.

The fact that your wife now knows that life will never be the same for her or your family is devastating. She will reflect on her past accomplishments and her dreams and goals for the future. This realization and reflection add fuel to the fire as your wife tries to put the pieces of the puzzle together. Sadness and anger prevail and, again, this is a normal response to a devastating and life-changing event, especially in the case of being diagnosed with multiple sclerosis.

Dr. Kubler-Ross goes on to say that "the grieving person may then be furious at the person who inflicted the hurt, or at the world, for letting it happen." In our case, I was to take the brunt of Martha's anger. She blamed me for her MS. Back in 2001, when I left Practice Administration in healthcare, I partnered with a colleague in a business venture that went sour within six months. I was bleeding financially. This debt burden caused a tremendous amount of stress on the family, especially on Martha.

Studies have shown that stress is not good for MS and can cause a relapse. Martha felt strongly that my business venture put her over the edge and "caused her MS to come out." Technically, she was correct. But for her to personally blame me was also difficult to accept. I would retort, "So I gave you the defective MS gene and told you where to live so you may be exposed to MS, right?"

Your wife will have a mix of emotions at this early stage since she is trying to cope with accepting the fact that she has MS. So, the first hurdle that your wife must overcome is to accept the onslaught of MS and to understand its impact on her life. But before she can fully accept that she has MS, she MUST experience this grief cycle.

Life is changing quickly, but it is not over by any means. Changes will occur and adaptation will be necessary, but you both can rise above it to new heights. Once the denial and anger phases have taken their course, your wife will enter the bargaining phase.

During the bargaining phase, your wife will realize that life has now changed regardless of her attitude. All that she can do in order to accept that she has MS is to believe in herself and her support group (in this case, YOU). She may try to bargain with God in various ways, but it does not change the outcome. Martha had a relatively short bargaining phase.

The fact that Martha knew she was now changed forever and could not do all the things she used to be able to do depressed her. Depression is the fourth stage in the grief cycle. Once Martha realized that her "old life" was over and that she HAD to move on, she was able to release the anger but this led to depression. It was a big step to accept that MS was now her sidekick for the rest of her life. She was required to learn new limitations and to be the master of her energy level. She realized quickly that energy was now her primary concern.

Acknowledging that she could no longer work full-time, Martha initiated the necessary steps to go out on disability leave. It was the best decision she made.

Martha was accustomed to a flurry of activity in the workplace and at home. She was one of six children in her family. Daily wrangles always occurred at "Camp Hillsdale." (She lived on Hillsdale Road in Lynchburg.) We nicknamed it this because her parents had to run their family like a boot camp.

The transition from full time work to going out on disability leave was a huge step for Martha to climb. "What am I going to do with my time?" she would ask. Knowing that she would have to find a part-time job in order to stave off depression was in and of itself depressing.

After six months of wrestling with such life-changing decisions, Martha was able to finally accept that she did have MS and could handle this disease. This acceptance occurred during the next six months. It was a gradual transition. Each day, Martha seemed to make more headway and was able to pull out of her depressed state. Finding the appropriate anti-depressant drug was also instrumental. It was all purely trial and error. She had to try three different drugs in order to finally find the best one for her.

Martha began taking Wellbutrin. She was also taking Amantadine for energy to combat fatigue. After about a year; however, she developed a rash. It appeared like a snakeskin where you could see the webbing in her veins. It was really weird. So she had to give up taking Amantadine and was prescribed Ritalin instead.

When she switched to this drug, Martha also changed her antidepressant to Effexor, but gave up this drug quickly. The sexual side effects were too severe. Instead, Martha was prescribed Lexapro, and she has been taking this drug ever since. Lexapro is both an antidepressant and an anti-anxiety medication. Thus, it is important to find the best combination of medication that represents the proper balance for your wife. Depression and fatigue are two of the most significant mental and physical hurdles your wife will have to overcome in her struggles with multiple sclerosis.

In retrospect, I believe the anger phase is the most trying phase of all. It is during this phase that your wife is experiencing a myriad of emotional and physical shifts. You have to remain strong and supportive. Understanding what she is battling will help you cope with this dynamic yet volatile period.

Chapter 5

IMPACT OF MS ON YOUR MARRIAGE

Since 2004, we have adjusted to life with MS. It has not been easy though, especially during that first year when Martha was first diagnosed. Sadly, many couples get divorced when a spouse is afflicted with MS. It is a big commitment to become a caregiver and a tremendous uncertainty does exist. Your vows for "in sickness and in health..." will surely be tested now that your wife has MS.

I have been married to my wife for twenty-eight years. I am blessed. Marriage is not easy. Add MS to the mix and you have yourself a dandy. But the good news is that you will come out of this major, life-changing event stronger than when you first encountered it. You are both in this together. You MUST remain by your wife's side and become her strongest advocate. She is going to rely on you more and more for both mental and physical support. Additionally, keep in mind that when your wife has MS, your whole family is affected.

Luckily for us, our kids were teenagers when MS started to rear its ugly head with Martha. They understood what was happening, but at the same time, I think they were also scared. Both girls were reluctant to talk openly about it. Conversations were strained often times so Martha and I just tried to reassure them that they had only a four percent chance of becoming afflicted with MS, due to genetics.

My heart goes out to those couples with young children. That situation presents more of a physical challenge since your wife will be combating fatigue and the children just do not understand why Mommy cannot go play with them all the time. When we are sad about Martha having MS, we quickly flip that sadness into joy when we focus on God's blessing that we had already raised our children by the time she was relapsing with MS.

To a certain extent, a role shift needs to occur in your marriage in order to maintain a healthy relationship, given the new pressures MS brings to the scene. I had already started to dabble in cooking, watching the food network shows. I would experiment with meals and cook on the weekends.

When Martha was diagnosed, I quickly realized that she did not have the energy to cook for the family anymore, let alone to go the grocery store. So I willingly accepted the role of grocery shopper, meal planner and chef. I made it fun. I started clipping coupons and made it a game to see how much I could save at Kroger by making a list of items to buy and seeing what I could get on sale and with a coupon.

Martha and the girls all enjoyed my cooking. My family ate well. I would always try to cook with fresh ingredients, using herbs and spices versus cream sauces etc. I usually do not follow recipes. I just throw together ingredients I know mix well together. The results are always positive. I try to cook enough for leftovers to take to work for my lunch the next day.

I remember when Elizabeth, my oldest daughter, was a senior in high school. She worked at a local restaurant a few nights a week as a waitress. She would come home late and often ate my Tupperware container with my lunch for the next day. After a few events like this, I started to put a note on it labeled "DAD'S LUNCH!"

Frequently, the kids' friends would stop by and partook of leftovers and they remarked how tasty they were. They are words a chef loves to hear.

Exercise also plays an important role in our life. We are both walkers. I became an avid walker when Martha was diagnosed in 2004. It is extremely important that you realize the many mental and physical benefits of exercise. You are encouraged to take a lead role in ensuring that your wife stays physically and mentally fit.

Your wife is constantly battling depression, so I suggest that you find an activity that you both enjoy, and one that you will "do" as a daily routine. For us, it is easy because we have a dog. Each day when I got home from work, we walked our dog Belle. In the summer heat, we had to adjust our route to one with more shade and Martha had to wear her cooling vest. On some days, it was just too hot and humid for her to walk anytime other than in the morning. So she would walk Belle in the morning and I walked alone after work.

In 2008, I trained for my fourth MS Challenge Walk. These MS Challenge Walks began for us one day in the spring of 2004 when I returned home from work and Martha informed me that she registered us for the fifty-mile walk that September. I was taken aback a bit, but I accepted the challenge. Right then, I decided that I would use this opportunity to really get into shape. Walking is a great exercise especially when you walk for, at least, several miles a day. Cardiologists have proven that, at least, thirty minutes of brisk walking daily is extremely beneficial to lowering your risk for cardiovascular problems. Walking is also a great stress reliever; you are outside experiencing nature and absorbing natural Vitamin D. When I walk, I talk to God, myself and my dog. Only on five-mile walks or longer would I use my IPOD. Otherwise, I enjoy hearing the sounds of other dogs barking, birds chirping and squirrels chattering away as they tease the dogs.

To a certain extent, your activities will need to change if you want to spend time together. Martha and I used to love to go boating, but now she is sensitive to the heat. MS and heat do not mix well. That first year, Martha and I made it a point to go to McArthur Mall on Friday nights and walk around in the coolness, and, sometimes, we would grab a bite to eat at a new restaurant on Granby Street. These Friday night "dates" were often preludes to a "shot night." We enjoyed the outing and the exercise, and it was always fun to "people-watch" at the mall when we rested. Martha and I find it fascinating to observe people and their interactions with each other and in groups.

Martha would say, "OK, find someone who looks kind of like me and point her out; someone with the same body size and pretty legs."

It is equally important for you to encourage your wife to explore her own hobbies if she does not already have one. These hobbies should also be something that she can

46

do alone or with another girlfriend. I find it necessary for me to still retain and maintain my "alone time." My alone time is spent fishing, gardening, and playing golf. It is important that you DO NOT give up your hobbies. You may merely compromise on the time you devote to your hobbies to care for your wife. If you do give up your hobbies to care for her, resentment will build inside you and that is not healthy.

Battling fatigue has been one of the most difficult situations for Martha. It angers her that she gets so tired. One of the ways she has learned to cope with decreased energy is to roll with it. She spends more time reading, taking naps, and writing notes. Note-writing is truly one of her God-given talents or gifts. She is expedient about sending nice cards and pictures to our friends after an event where she has taken a lot of pictures. Usually within twenty-four hours, the pictures have been printed and either hand-delivered or mailed with a thoughtful card.

Whether it is a sympathy card or a birthday card, Martha is always brightening someone's day with her notes. The time she spends picking out a special card and then writing a thoughtful note is uplifting for the receiver. The fact that someone thought enough about them to take the time to pick out a card, and write a note means a lot to people.

Lastly, your wife will most likely want to get heavily involved with one or several MS initiatives, and she will expect some of your time as well. Please willingly accept and embrace the causes your wife chooses to get involved in. She needs to feel passionate about something, for she has been stripped off a part of her life by being diagnosed with MS.

For us, Martha's passion is being a patient advocate for Biogen Idec. Biogen Idec's Patient Advocate program interested Martha. This is a program where patients can learn how present their story of MS and inspire other MS patients at drug company-sponsored programs. Usually, a patient advocate would be present with a physician during the two-hour program on a Tuesday or Thursday evening, or, sometimes, on Saturday mornings. The key is that Martha became involved in a cause early on. Otherwise, she would have become depressed as many patients do once they have been diagnosed and try to survive while undergoing all the life-changing processes.

She first spoke about her experiences on Avonex and, since 2006; she speaks about her experiences on Tysabri. She was involved with a group called Patients for Choice. This advocacy group organized an effort to petition the FDA to hold an advisory board meeting when Tysabri was pulled from the market and was planning to be re-introduced. She testified in front of the FDA on March 7, 2005.

The people you meet with MS are diverse and dynamic. Their stories vary from hope and encouragement to disappointment and disability. When Martha testified in front of the FDA, I had the opportunity to be present for this significant yet highly emotional event. At this hearing, forty-four Tysabri patients each were allotted three minutes to present their testimony to the advisory board. When your three minutes were up, they cut the volume to the microphone.

I helped Martha write her speech and we timed it over and over again. She was right on the money.

I would have to say that people with MS, and their spouses and families, are some of the finest individuals you will ever know. They have experienced loss, heartache and disappointment yet they are strong, hopeful and faithful.

Chapter 6

RELY ON YOUR FAITH

It has been said that the true measure of a person is not in how many times they get knocked down, but how many times they rise up after the fall. It is your response to adversity that matters. You can be able to cope with adversity and emerge from it even stronger than you were, if you have a strong faith. Your trust in Christ, who lives within you, enables you to adapt and learn how to live a full life, despite having a disease or another adversity that challenges you. Just take one quick look at people with terminal cancer, especially the sweet children. Most of them are content and feel protected and blessed because of their strong beliefs. They have found peace through accepting their situation and knowing that God loves them and they are finally going "home." Long ago, I stopped questioning God with "Why did this happen to me?" or "Why did this happen to my wife?"

You just have to accept the situation for what it is. Life is full of so many mysteries that we cannot explain. As Forest Gump reminds us in his movie, "Life is like a box of chocolates; you never know what you're going to get until you bite into it." That is where your faith comes in. Webster defines <u>faith</u> as: *belief and trust in and loyalty to God: belief in the traditional doctrines of a religion: firm belief in something for which there is no proof: complete trust.*

It is our beliefs that form our faith, and we are exposed to denominational beliefs through our faith communities. Over time, our faith grows as we nurture it by attending worship services, by reading and studying the Bible, and by praying.

Luckily for me, my parents brought me up in the church. I was raised a Methodist. They made us go to Sunday school and church every week. As a kid, you sort of hate it, at first; because you are being forced to go, but after a while, it becomes a part of you. I thank my parents for baptizing me when I was an infant and for bringing me into the church. It is extremely important to worship God by attending a church community and becoming involved in the activities, especially after baptism and confirmation. My parents belonged to Epworth United Methodist Church where I attended until I was married.

My wife was raised a Catholic and she is from Lynchburg. She was baptized and confirmed at Holy Trinity Church. She attended mass with her family regularly. Regular mass attendance was mandatory in her family and she and her siblings also attended Catholic schools when they were in elementary and middle school grades.

When I met Martha and we discussed religion, it was clear that she would remain Catholic and our kids should be raised Catholic. I had no problems with that. Since meeting her, we attended Catholic mass. I was intrigued by the rituals and the participation of the congregation during the worship service. Over the years, I learned the responses but I remained a Methodist. I called myself a practicing Catholic and remarked to my wife, "I do not need to convert. I am a Christian and a Methodist. Converting to Catholicism will not change how I worship God, neither will it change my relationship with God."

Oh well! I did convert in April 2000, totally of my own volition. I thank Martha for never pressuring me. After attending Sacred Heart Catholic Church in Ghent in Norfolk for fifteen years, I felt I needed to become a full member of this parish community. I attended the RCIA program which is the Rite of Christian Initiation for Adults. This program began in August and continued through the following Easter when I was confirmed. The Catholic faith recognizes any church who baptizes in the name of the Father, Son and Holy Ghost. Those candidates only need to be confirmed.

Since becoming Catholic, my faith has grown tremendously. I truly believe that the focus on the Liturgy and the Eucharist in the Catholic Church has changed me. The nourishment of Eucharist every week and the understanding of its meaning for our lives is reinforced constantly. I am most thankful that God was crafting my life to this point where I was well-grounded in my faith. I firmly believe that my confidence in HIM, that Martha will prevail in this battle with MS, has afforded me the strength and the attitude to be an understanding caregiver to my wife.

You must be able to console and comfort her, to uplift her when she is down; but you also have to be strong enough to challenge her and rein her in when the going gets tough and she wants to fall back into the "blame game and woe is me" mentality. That is a common and expected phenomenon. As a caregiver, you have to be prepared to effectively handle this situation. If not addressed properly, you may, instead of aiding your wife, actually feed her with anxiety which will then fuel her depression.

Numerous times, I found myself consoling Martha in that first six months. I had to reassure her often, saying, "Honey, it could've been worse; you could've had cancer. At least, with MS, you won't die."

She would respond angrily, "Yeah, but you don't have MS, now do you? I do and it sucks."

On several occasions, I have conversed with Martha about her afflictions and suffering since she would frequently retort, "Why do I have to have this disease? Haven't I been through enough in my life already?"

I would have to remind her of Job's afflictions. We do not understand why one suffers more than another. Yet it is not our right to question God and to blame God for these afflictions. We cannot comprehend them because we are finite beings. All that we can do is to learn to deal with the deck of cards that have been given to us, as I like to say. It is our response to adversity that makes a difference.

During the extremely challenging moments, we prayed together about this disease. I lift Martha up in prayer daily and thank God for how well she is doing. I know Martha prays similarly. I give thanks to God for truly blessing Martha with good health. I know it could be a LOT worse. I have seen it first hand at many MS functions. I have seen people on walkers, in wheel chairs and in scooters. I remember how excited one lady whom we met was. We called her the 'scooter lady." She was so proud of her new scooter. I admired her for finding joy despite her disability. Martha would observe this, however, and say, "I am not going to end up like that."

I would agree with her, but would say to myself, "I certainly hope and pray you won't either." There are no certainties in this life, other than death and taxes, and the only certain thing about MS is the uncertainty of how this disease can progress and how it affects everyone differently. It is a puzzling disease; however, our wonderful physicians and researchers are beginning to understand its multi-symptom nature.

As mentioned earlier in this book, only when your wife has fully accepted her new condition, can she move on and begin to adjust to new changes in her life. Her faith in God may be strained during this time, however, it will prevail. To fully trust God is one of the most challenging aspects of our daily lives.

I now, more than ever before, cherish the beauty and gift of each day, with all its challenges and opportunities presented. My motto is "Carpe Diem." The bible tells us to be joyful and hopeful, to be diligent in our prayers and our faith. I am always reassured when I read the verse from Matthew 6:26 that states: *"Look at the birds of the air; they do not sow, nor reap nor gather into barns, and yet your heavenly Father feeds them. Are you not worth much more than they?"*

My favorite Scriptural verses are from Philippians 4:6-7. These verses say:

"6. Be anxious for nothing, but in everything by prayer and supplication with thanksgiving let your requests be made known to God.

"7. And the peace of God, which surpasses all comprehension, will guard your hearts and your minds in Christ Jesus."

To me, these verses of the Scriptures sum up my faith. God does not want us to worry; He wants us to be thankful and to pray about everything. If we do our part, by spending time with God and by praying about our concerns faithfully, then He will bless us and answer our prayers. I do not mean, He will "do it for you"; rather, God will show you the way and infuse you with His power and strength to endure your challenges.

The key here is to understand that the ensuing peace which will come over you cannot be completely understood. God is infinite and beyond human comprehension. We believe in the Trinity, yet we cannot fully explain or understand it. It is that peace that unites us with Jesus, heart and soul. Our brains are very powerful organs. Too often, we humans fail to harness its power.

I was seventeen when I learned those verses. They captivated me at the time and I realized then that worry and anxiety are not good for one's health. I was active in the Young Life program in high school. Young Life was a bible study group for high school kids. We would meet weekly and were involved with other groups who would travel to Young Life functions throughout the country to youth camps and be volunteers on the work crew.

One of my most memorable experiences was when I was a freshman in college. I met this girl named Laura Wolf. We became great friends and both of us had an opportunity with Young Life of America to go to Lake Saranac in New York to be part of the work crew for a week. The camp site was beautiful and there were probably about three hundred high school kids there. Our primary duties were to assist with preparing meals in the kitchen.

It was an awesome experience to serve these kids. God blessed us as we had time to engage in mini spiritual retreats. To be alone with God, meditating and praying in such a beautiful place along the Lake was inspirational and gratifying. Yes, we were tired but God gave us the strength to perform our duties.

As Napoleon Hill contends in his book <u>Think and Grow Rich</u>; many extremely successful people do not have extraordinary talent; what they do have is an incredible *burning desire* to succeed. One takes that burning desire and turns it into well thought out plans of action. These plans, coupled with an intense commitment to NEVER give up trying until you have reached your goal, is the key to extreme success. Imagine what happens if we applied these secular attributes to our spiritual lives? Look at what Jesus did for us. He had a burning desire to die for all of humanity's sins. Let us allow Him to ignite our burning desire so that we can carry out His mission here on earth to bring forth His kingdom.

Accepting that she now has MS was burdensome for Martha from the onset. She had endured many trials and tribulations during the nineties. In 1994, she ruptured two discs in her neck and had to have surgery to have these discs fused together. They used cadaver bone to implant in the ruptured disc and then fused them together. She fully recovered but this was still a very traumatic event.

In 1999, Bernie, her father, died of prostate cancer. She was in graduate school then, pursuing her degree at Old Dominion University to become a teacher. She was working part-time at Norfolk Collegiate lower school, since Sarah was in fourth grade. Looking back on this period, I wonder now if this was not the first clinical signs of MS starting to emerge in Martha's life. It seemed she was overwhelmed and her concentration was clearly affected. The stress of the situation interfered with her cognitive abilities. With only six hours left to complete the graduate program, Martha decided against pursuing her degree; she had too much going on in her life and the death of her father was devastating.

I believe that Bernie's strong spirit has assisted Martha in living with MS. Martha was very close to her father and knows that his spirit lives on in her. Bernie always pushed the envelope, so to speak. He never quitted. A common saying in his family was "no quitters in this family."

Much in the same way, Martha pushes herself everyday living with MS. To others, she makes it look easy, but it is not by any means easy. I know for certain that God has blessed Martha with excellent health, despite having MS. It is clear to me now how He is guiding her to be an inspiration to others. Martha inspires others through the Patient Advocate talks and through just plain living. She is so positive and lights up any room. Martha can start a conversation with any stranger, whether it is at the grocery store or on an elevator. Her bright smile just warms peoples' hearts immediately.

We watched the movie called the Celestine Prophecy a few years ago. What I remember most about the movie I also find to be true about people and relationships. We each have an "aura" about us; this is our physical, spiritual and emotional energy. This energy is either positive or negative. Positive energy is that which freely flows out of one person into another to build them up. Negative energy is that energy which "sucks out" any positive energy from the other person, acting as a drain on the positive person's energy.

I have found that this phenomenon holds true in most circumstances in life when you meet people. Those you surround yourself with either pick you up emotionally, or drain your energy. Individuals who are generally positive will certainly experience hardship and challenges. They need your support during these times. One gladly and freely gives positive emotional support (physical energy) to that person to help lift their spirits up. And the person freely giving this positive energy is uplifted in the process.

In contrast, when you are surrounded by people who are primarily negative and downtrodden, they tend to drain you without you getting anything in return. Keep in mind, though; we do need to be kind and loving to others and offer support even when it drains us, but not all the time. For example, when Martha was first diagnosed with MS, she attended an MS Support group locally. She arrived home several hours later more depressed than when she left. Martha remarked, "Everyone there was just 'Woe is me!' It was depressing! I am never going back there. I don't need that kind of support!"

So Martha turned to the internet and began researching MS and she learned that the drug company Biogen Idec, offered a program for patients with MS called the Patient Advocate Program. This program provided her the opportunity to meet others with MS who are coping with MS exceptionally well and have a positive outlook and are inspirational.

Through the patient advocate program, Martha and I have met some truly outstanding individuals. Each person has his or her own story to reveal. MS affects everyone differently. Martha and the other advocates are blessed; they have overcome numerous obstacles and learned to live a quality life despite having MS.

Living with MS is a difficult adjustment and Martha has been able to cope with this disease. I know that the strong faith community at Sacred Heart and their prayers catapulted Martha to the next level.

I remember when Martha finally accepted MS and was deeply involved with the Advocate training program and corresponding with the Biogen representatives and other MS patients. She told me then, "I want to become the MS poster child. I am going to do it."

Right then, I knew she would achieve this goal and, today, she is one of about one hundred seasoned Patient Advocates. Martha's ultimate acceptance of MS arrived in August 2006 when Tysabri had been re-introduced to the market and she was able to resume her monthly infusions. She had suffered a major setback when it was pulled from the market in February 2005. Tysabri, I feel, provides Martha with the physical and mental strength to persevere and to hold back MS from preventing any further damage to her brain and/or spinal column.

By its nature, Tysabri blocks the T cells from entering the brain. So in many respects, Tysabri does make patients better since it stops MS from even getting into the brain. Furthermore, I am confident that Martha's positive outlook on her life is significantly aided by knowing that this drug really does its job well. It is the most effective drug to treat relapsing-remitting MS in the market today. Fortunately, we have great health insurance through my company and her Medicare Part B, which pays for the costs of this treatment.

Chapter 7

TEAM SACRED HEART – CHALLENGE YOURSELF

Our faith and involvement with our church Sacred Heart Catholic Church in Ghent in Norfolk, Virginia, provided us with a firm foundation to face life's many challenges. The situations I described in Chapter Three during Martha's initial diagnosis would have been disastrous if it were not for the strong faith community at our church supporting my family during my absence. Those first few months are always the scariest, and here I was being called out of town by my job for three months.

Martha was spending time on the internet searching for information and community involvement with MS. She tried a local support group early on, but it was not for her. She returned home more depressed than when she left. So right then, she decided that she would choose other ways to get involved.

She signed up for email from the local Hampton Roads Chapter. Martha also visited their web site. The local chapter web site was a wealth of information, detailing upcoming patient education programs, the latest updates on treatment options, and scheduled events. I remember her calling me in late February telling me about the MS five-mile walk that was scheduled for Virginia Beach in May 2004.

She was still in the early stages of coming to grips with this disease and remarked that it was a good cause to participate in, but she was in no condition to raise money and walk in a few months at this event. Besides, she was still unsteady on her feet, so we decided we would participate in the walk the following year. Our immediate need was to get this disease under control and to learn to cope with daily challenges of fatigue, depression, balance and gait issues. She was still working full-time, which made it even more of an uphill battle. Plus, I was still out of town and life was absolutely crazy.

We decided that a focus on fitness was paramount. When I returned home in April, we started walking a mile or so in the neighborhood. I had to hold her hand and we had to walk real slowly. Martha was still scared about what was happening to her. I reassured her that she was strong and she could weather this frightening storm.

Gradually, Martha's strength increased but her balance was still off. She decided on physical therapy as a treatment option in order to regain her balance and strength. She began physical therapy in April of 2004. The practice was called North Shore Sports and Physical Therapy. It was convenient and Lisa Koperna, her therapist, was truly amazing.

Lisa worked with Martha for about three to four months, assisting her in regaining balance and core strength. I witnessed much progress in her therapy. Additionally, these visits were mentally therapeutic as Lisa encouraged Martha once she learned her life story. Lisa thought Martha was amazing to be doing so well with this disease, despite a few balance issues. Lisa often said, after hearing Martha's stories, "You should write a book." Well, we are; I just happen to be the author telling Martha's story!

When the e-mail arrived about the five-mile walk in 2005, I decided right then that Martha and I would join the ranks of fellow MS'ers in this walk at Virginia Beach. It took me only a few minutes to decide to participate as a team and the name of our team would be Team Sacred Heart, in honor of our church. Team Sacred Heart was well-represented in the spring of 2005 with twenty-eight walkers. The five-mile MS walk was held annually at Virginia Beach and Newport News, Virginia. I felt strongly that we needed to support the MS community by getting involved, raising some money, walking five miles and meeting others who faced our same dilemma. The local MS Society provided us with great tools to launch a fundraising effort via e-mail and letters. In total, we had twenty-eight team members and collectively raised $4,800.

Our friends at church rallied around us and Martha's neurologist, Tom Pellegrino, and his wife also joined us for the walk. His best friends, Annette and Gene Field also joined us. We did not know them very well at the time. I remember receiving a check in the mail from Annette Field for $100 and not really knowing who she was. A beautiful and inspirational note was with the check. On the day of the walk, we realized who she was. We all went to the same mass and so we recognized Gene Field and Annette Field once we saw them.

Several other very important people to Martha participated in this walk. Will King, headmaster of Norfolk Collegiate School (NCS), was a member of our team. Other NCS team members included Christy Sykes, a teacher; Jack Kavanaugh, a board member; and another board member who had MS. She was in a wheelchair, and Will King pushed her for five miles down the boardwalk.

Many other friends joined us, along with my two teenage daughters, Elizabeth and Sarah. They were not too happy about being up so early on a Sunday morning but were with us to support Martha. My sisters had previous commitments and were unable to join us.

My cousin, Dr. Gordon Stokes, and his wife Kerri participated as well. He is a vascular surgeon and she is a pediatrician. As healthcare providers, they were keenly interested in our cause. My good friend from long ago, Randall Greene, flew in from Florida to join our team. That meant a lot to me and proved what a great and true friend Randall was, and is to this day. Actions speak louder than words, and his trip to Norfolk was a testimony to that sentiment.

As always, Martha was prepared for the Kodak moment. She whipped out her camera and started telling us where to position ourselves for the team pictures. She recruited a bystander to take our pictures. After several series of group and mini-group pictures, we were ready to start walking. The majority of the money raised during walk campaigns like this one was dedicated to support research efforts to end multiple sclerosis.

Everyone gathered at the park on 31st street at the starting line. The route was from 31st street, down to Rudee Inlet and back up to 45th street, and then everyone returned to 31st street to the finish line. It was a blustery day, around 55 to 60 degrees Fahrenheit, but the sun was out. I had on several shirts since it was a bit chilly. Already sporting a bit of a belly, the extra shirts made it look even bigger!

I remember both Gordy and Randall commenting on my stomach. Now I am not that fat at all; I just have a large frame AND a large belly. At that moment, I was determined to start getting into better shape and lose the extra weight and belly fat. Walking became my passion from that moment on.

Several thousand people were present at this important event. Along the route, the society had posters with snippets of relevant facts about MS. While walking, we met others much less fortunate than us. When you see a young husband pushing his wife in a wheelchair and the two young kids in tow behind him, it gives you a much better perspective of your own situation and makes life look pretty good at that point. We realized, then, that MS could be much worse for Martha.

I remember clearly the concern and fear in Martha's demeanor when she saw many young people afflicted with MS. This is the devastating aspect of this disease. MS does not discriminate; young or old, it all depends on when you had your initial attack and at what stage MS first attacks your body. In some individuals, the impact of MS on their motor and speech functions is extremely severe and rapid. For most people, in the last ten years, drug therapy has been available to treat even the most aggressive symptoms. However, not everyone has health insurance. And for those who do, the drug therapy is not cheap either.

I could see the "reality check" in Martha's expression as I held her hand and she, Randall and I walked down the boardwalk. Our pace was slower than our friends, since Martha was still slightly unsteady on her feet so I had to hold her hand most of the time. And I had not seen Randall in about five or six years, so it was nice for him to walk with us so we could catch up on our lives.

Most of the walkers had finished the five-mile walk in about two hours. They allowed enough time for those walking slowly to complete the walk. I remember how impressed I was by a certain black lady who was probably in her early sixties. Clearly, she had MS. She methodically completed the walk, every step of the way, with the assistance of her cane. Even though Martha's gait was unsteady at times, she had my hand to hold onto. She remarked several times that day, "I am not going to end up with a cane or in a wheelchair."

I would console her and agree, all the while respecting her heartfelt strength and determination to fight this disease head on, but, at the same time, realizing that many uncertainties exist with having MS. One never knows what is going to happen next. This is why we embrace the joys of each day, since good health with MS is truly a blessing for Martha and our family. Things could be a lot worse! I know they could.

At the finish line, under a tent, they had food and drinks for us. There was pizza and subway sandwiches and cookies. Our friends from church hung out for a while, conversing on the boardwalk. The fellowship we enjoyed with friends and family on the boardwalk after completing the five-mile walk was rejuvenating. The weather was perfect. The bright sun was out, the waves were breaking and the pelicans were gliding just above the waves, as they rolled along the coast.

The overall message of the day was one of hope. Support for individuals with MS is strong. Organizations like the local Hampton Roads Chapter of the National Multiple Sclerosis Society strive to educate patients and providers on the most effective methods to treat this disease. They sponsor events like this to raise money for research efforts and to host educational programs.

They had a booth set up called the "Challenge Booth." Sharon Grossman, the Hampton Roads MS chapter president at that time, was stationed at the booth and I remember her pressing us to "take the challenge" and to sign up for the fifty-mile walk. She had walked the fifty miles the prior year and presented us with a convincing argument. I remember thinking to myself, "Fifty miles in three days? That is a challenge!" Martha also heard this challenge. If you know my wife, you'll understand that she also loves a challenge. She has an ingrained sense to constantly push herself. This seed was now firmly planted in her mind about the MS Challenge Walk.

A month later, in early June, I arrived home from work one day to hear that Martha had signed us up for the fifty-mile walk in October in Maryland. I retorted, "OK," kind of hesitantly, since she had not consulted me prior to plunking down $55 per person for the privilege of walking fifty miles but that wasn't all:

"Oh, by the way," she said, "We each must raise $1,500.00 minimum, in order to walk."

At first, the thought of each of us raising that sum of money did seem a bit daunting. However, I tried to focus on the health benefits that would be derived from training for the fifty-miler. I reassured myself that we were both seasoned sales people and could rely on our network of family and friends to join our cause and contribute. The web page developed for the MS Challenge Walk hosted a variety of tools such as a sample fundraising letter and instructions for how to easily customize your own web page. My first steps were to complete both my web page and Martha's, and then complete the fundraising letter. The next step was to make a list of all our friends so we would not duplicate our efforts.

Once you make a list of ALL the people you know, the task seems much less daunting. Your $1,500 can be raised in no time since most people will, at least, give you $25 which will equate to a total of sixty (60) donations if you only receive an average of $25. Factor in your family and really close friends, and your averages increase since you will receive frequent donations of $50 from close friends and $100 or $200 donations from family members. A reasonable mix of donations average out to about 40 donors at most, with the combinations above.

E-mail is an incredibly efficient but less personal method of fund-raising. Our experience has been that approximately fifteen percent of those folks you email will actually donate online or bother to send you a check in the mail. Our preferred method of raising money for MS is the "SASE" method. SASE stands for Self Addressed Stamped Envelope. This is where you print off a letter and write a brief personal note on it, and include a stamped, return envelope. I used to put one of my return address labels as the addressee on the envelope so, literally, all the person had to do was write a check, put it in your envelope provided and attach their own return address label, and then drop it in the mail.

Your success with this method will be outstanding. You can always follow up with a phone call and joke with them, "I need my envelope back with the stamp to pay a bill if you don't send me a check!" Most people will donate after this soft ribbing. I have only had one person not donate with this method.

Collectively, Martha and I raised a total of $3,900 that first year. We won an award for our combined fundraising efforts for 2005. With the five-mile walk and the fifty-mile walk, our team, Team Sacred Heart, raised a total of approximately $9,300. We were pleased with our efforts and gladly accepted the reward at the local chapter meeting.

Fund-raising is not the most important aspect of this cause though. When a person makes a commitment to walk the MS Challenge Walk, it serves as a motivator, showing determination, and a focused interest to be involved with the cause for the fight against MS. Approximately 20% of the individuals who participate in these walks have MS. A secondary benefit from the Challenge Walk is, of course, the exercise component.

Staying fit will promote one's ability to stave off some of the effects of MS.

Once I read the materials on the web page about the type of clothing we should wear for the walks, we made a trip to Running Etc. to purchase shoes and to Sports Authority to buy our clothes and socks. It is critical that your socks contain no cotton. "Cotton is rotten." Once cotton gets soaked with sweat, it promotes blisters. Therefore, you must purchase 'wicking' socks which contain no fibers. Go ahead and spend the $7 to $12 per pair of socks. And you need at least 3 pairs. We also purchased wicking shorts, shirts and underwear. Including the purchase of our shoes, between the two of us, we probably spent $300 on the proper clothing that first year. This was money well spent. Do not scrimp on your shoes either. You MUST have the proper equipment for the job at hand.

We liked the staff at our local running store, Running Etc., since they were knowledgeable and would work with you to ensure the proper fit and type of shoe. Most advise purchasing a standard running shoe for the long MS Challenge Walk. The staff will advise you to get a shoe at least a half size larger than your normal shoe size; your foot will swell on long walks so you need the extra length. And it is important to be sized for the right width of shoe also. I have a wide foot so it is more difficult for me to find shoes that fit.

I had purchased a pair of Saucony's the previous year and found them to fit well. I decided I would try the same brand and Running Etc. had the brand but not my previous year's model. This is typical. I purchased the current model which had a bit wider toe box. I walked two miles or so daily in order to break them in.

I noticed a change in my stride and felt my right foot was "clopping" down rather than a smooth heel to toe stride. After a week, I knew something was not right. I had developed pain in my right ankle, shin and calf. This pain was from the darn shoes. I quickly returned them for a pair of Asics, which I have continued to purchase each year since.

Worse yet, this pain was so bad that I had to start physical therapy! I was concerned to be in physical therapy this close to the walk. We had ramped up our training and were walking eight miles on Saturday mornings. The pain was so bad that after 1.5 miles, my right leg just burned for about the next 4.5 miles and did not stop hurting until mile six. This pain persisted for three weeks, so needless to say the Saturday morning walks were painful, literally. But thanks to Miss Lisa, she performed a combination of heat and ultrasound massage therapy on my leg along with prescribed stretching exercises. I practiced these at home and eventually the pain subsided.

During these early morning walks, Martha wore her cooling vest since she was sensitive to the heat. In the summer of 2004, we purchased a cooling vest that was lightweight but was activated in water. These "cells" hydrated. You then wrung out the vest before wearing it. Martha was a real sport about it. The vest worked OK, but at the time, we did not have $100 we could spend on a more effective vest.

Martha amazed me how she could walk six to eight miles in the summer heat during training for the MS Challenge Walk. I could see the results of her months in physical therapy. Her balance was steady, her gait much smoother and I did not have to hold her hand until the last few miles. I would listen for the sound of her foot dropping and without saying a word, would just put out my hand which she gladly took.

As team captain, I organized our early morning walks with our other team mates. Our team was comprised of Martha, myself, Nancy King and Anne Richardson. We varied our Saturday morning routes; one week we would walk in our neighborhood and the following week, their neighborhood. We felt energized by the end of our walks. Most folks are just waking up and still drinking coffee at 9:15 in the morning, but here we were, having just completed an invigorating eight mile walk!

During late July through early September, we increased our walking distance to nine and ten miles and we also completed a few twelve mile walks in preparation for the fifty-miler in October. Martha was able to walk the eight miles on Saturday mornings but was unable to walk any further.

Approximately three weeks before the date of the Challenge Walk, she started complaining that both big toes were really hurting and it was more difficult for her to walk longer distances. Upon closer examination, we found that she had bruised her big toes so much that the nails were falling off.

I clearly remember the Saturday morning at the Podiatrist's office up the road from our house when she called me and asked me to come hold her hand as she was about to be injected so the doctor could cut out the nails since they had not completely fallen off. My wife is one tough lady. But that was an extremely painful and unpleasant experience. It hurt me just to watch the procedure.

We deduced that Martha's toes were longer than normal and her shoes were not long enough. This close to the walk, however, was not enough time to purchase new shoes and break them in. We determined that she would not walk longer than five miles at any one clip and she would survive without any further damage to her toes. This episode is just one of many examples of Martha's resilience with this disease. Challenges just keep coming her way and she gracefully accepts them head on and usually overcomes them, although with some level of pain and suffering. Having MS is not easy.

As the Challenge Walk date approached, we all felt well-trained for the walk. I was very proud of Martha and felt she was strong enough for the upcoming challenge. It was a daunting task to walk fifty miles in three days, but we rationalized that the first two days were simply two 10 mile segments. Or so we thought.

The first day of the walk, we congregated in a marina parking lot in Chester, Virginia on the eastern shore. It was a pleasant morning, and was actually warmer than usual, which concerned us. Our route was through neighborhoods and along a country road. They had rest stops every 2.5 miles with plenty of snacks and water and Gatorade and portable potties. I witnessed Martha's face starting to flush after about five miles. She was not wearing her cooling vest, as we thought it would not be so hot. She struggled through the next segment and I told her to get a ride in the Sports And Gear (SAG) car to the next rest area. She was tiring and I did not want her to get overheated. I told her I would catch up with her in a few miles.

The morning continued to get hotter and I was glad that Martha took a break from walking, to rest and let her core body temperature decrease a few degrees since she had clearly become overheated. We joined up with each other at about mile 12.5. She then walked with me to the stop at mile 14 for lunch. That was a welcome break.

After lunch, much to our surprise, they sent us back through some of the same route, which was quite hot and unpleasant. To make a long story short, Martha determined that the best method for her was to walk about 5 miles, then to sag for about 5 miles. I am so glad she employed this approach because the last part of the walk on the first day from mile 16 to 21.5 was horrible.

We had to walk through the neighborhood from hell, as we all named it. The asphalt was very rough and we were all tired and hot. Around mile 17.5, I experienced an excruciating pain in the arch of my left foot for about 10 seconds. It eventually subsided, but that scared me since it almost dropped me right to my knees. All in all, though, my feet were holding up pretty well. I was glad that I changed my socks out at lunch. I could feel a few hot spots developing on the balls of my feet, however.

We finished the first day and were then hoarded onto a bus for a thirty minute ride back to Camp Letts. Camp

Letts was a YMCA camp. As camps go, it was nice, but we slept in bunk beds, there was no A/C, bathrooms were community, and the food was OK. All I wanted was a few beers, but no alcohol was allowed. Gosh darn! After walking 21.5 miles, one deserves a beer or two! We showered up and rested before dinner, and then we all went to bed early. I knew I would have to attend to my feet the next morning, applying some mole skin for extra padding.

The route for the second day was much better. I kept telling myself that if I made it through the first day, the second day would not be so bad. But now having walked 21.5 miles, I knew I could do it again. Martha's plan on day two was to walk one segment of 2.5 miles, and then to sag to the next stop. I thought that made a lot of sense. She has MS and she doesn't need to push herself until she has a relapse. She was comfortable with not walking the whole fifty miles. The second day was much more enjoyable for all of us. The weather cooled down a bit and the course was a much easier route. Not having to walk along a country road with no shade at all made a huge difference.

Toward the end of the second day, I was jogging part of the way just to break up the monotony of walking so many miles. Also, running uses different sets of muscles so it helped me avoid cramping up. I would run for a quarter mile or so, walk some, and then run some more. I did not run too much though, since I could feel the hot spots getting warmer on my feet when I ran.

I was so excited to see my beautiful wife waiting for me at the finish line. She had a camera ready as I ran across it. I felt like I had accomplished so much by walking 40 miles in two days. Tomorrow would be a piece of cake, just having to walk ten miles total. Martha walked ten miles on Day One and ten miles on Day Two. Her feet were quite sore and she had a few blisters. We decided it would not be prudent for her to walk the final day.

On Day Three, she wore her sandals. We knew she could make that final one mile march to the auditorium at Baltimore's Inner Harbor in her sandals. That is exactly what she did. Our team picture at the pre-finish line shows her wearing her sandals. In total, Martha walked 21 miles. That is phenomenal for someone newly diagnosed with MS. I was so proud of her.

In 2006, our chapter changed the walk from a three-day, fifty-mile challenge, to a two-day, fifty-kilometer (50 KM) walk. This suited most folks much better. Our team trained again as we did the prior year. The only exception was that we started walking eight milers earlier in the summer and then extended them to 10 and 12 milers occasionally. We were in better shape the second year. Martha trained hard that year and, unfortunately, caught a horrible cold the week just before the Challenge Walk. She did not participate that year. It was not the same without her, but she made the correct decision.

I remember speaking at the candlelight ceremony, as a spouse of someone with MS. It brought tears to my eyes when I told the audience how much I loved my wife and how life changes when your spouse is diagnosed with MS.

In 2007, Anne Richardson was unable to walk with us, but Nancy King joined us. Martha's system was to walk one segment and then sag to the next rest stop. That really worked well for her and enabled her to meet many people along the way both walking and riding, and waiting for me to arrive at the next rest stop.

In 2008, we were lucky enough to recruit a new team member, Katie Daly. She and Martha walked together most of the time and Nancy and I walked together. Katie did not join our team till the end of the summer, so she had little time to train. However, she walked over 20 miles. She and Martha would walk and sag together, so it worked out well.

Knowing your own personal limits and the limits of your spouse are important. I knew that, personally, I WILL walk every inch of that 50KM while Martha's approach is, 'I will walk what I can. I am not going to push myself." I agreed with her. She was out there doing it and also did a phenomenal job of fundraising.

Chapter 8

YOUR ROLE AS HUSBAND & CAREGIVER

The most important aspect of being a caregiver is your mental toughness. Your wife is going to rely on you in ways you may or may not be accustomed to, or even want to accept. It is critical that you figure out quickly what your new role is going to be. It is unfortunate that in many marriages, when a spouse is diagnosed with MS, the structure of the marriage and household seems to crumble, and you hear of husbands who just don't seem to care, or even divorce their wives.

I think that is unconscionable. You are in the marriage together, for better or worse, till death. That is my philosophy. Understanding your wife's fatigue will help you adapt quickly to your new role, whether it be to help her vacuum the house, to cook meals or to do the grocery shopping. She just does not have the energy to perform these tasks like she used to. In our case, Martha was still working full-time.

She would arrive home from work and just have to get in bed. She was short-tempered and quite irritable, since she did not feel well. I thought to myself, "Boy, she is being mean to me. What have I done to her to deserve this kind of treatment?"

I dismissed this whiny attitude pretty shortly into the early stages, since you cannot take her outbursts personally. Anger and short-temperedness is a natural response when someone does not feel well and they are tired and have to push themselves so much. Martha literally pushed herself out of bed each day to get up and go to work and did it all over again on a daily basis. This grind took its toll on her so I knew I needed to help out.

The first role shift came in the cooking department. I was already enjoying watching the many Food Network cooking shows and started to experiment with different recipes. I discovered quickly that I had a natural knack for this and I enjoyed it immensely. So I told Martha, "From this point on, I am in charge of meal planning, grocery shopping and cooking. You and the kids can clean up dishes. I am not doing both." Cooking became my passion.

Meal planning takes a little time and effort. I always found that preparing a shopping list and having coupons was extremely helpful. One note about coupons, though; only save the ones that you will use. Don't buy a food item you do not regularly eat just because you have a coupon. The other thing I learned is that you have to price the store generic brands for Ziploc sandwich bags. For example; I found that the Kroger brands were just as good as Ziploc and cheaper even after the coupon, so why use it?

In our case, it was much easier to cook for four since we still had two teenage daughters at home. Besides, I enjoyed cooking a big meal so I had leftovers. I felt dedicated to this new cause, so I could bring a sense of stability to my family in an effort to help them cope with the changing family dynamics.

The second role shift was that of a life as a therapist. I had to listen to my wife deal with life-changing situations frequently, and she needed a sounding board. I would try my best to assimilate her anxieties, depressed moods, bouts of anger/acceptance and frustration, all wrapped into one neat package! As I mentioned earlier, the first year is the most difficult, as your spouse is coping with change. My best advice for you here is "not to take it personally." If she lashes out at you, it is not your fault. Just listen to her and try to redirect her emotions.

It is important for you to offer your spouse a "filtered" view of the situation. I learned a long time ago that somebody is always worse off than you. Remember the old adage, "When the going gets tough, the tough get going?" That holds true in this instance, in my opinion. Living with MS is a day by day event. You never know what tomorrow will bring you.

Your wife is going to have a very difficult adaptation period to her new life with MS, as will you; so it is important to talk to each other about how you will make adjustments to everyday living. Words like "I can only imagine how you must feel…." can be comforting.

The third role shift and one of the most important is that of a caregiver. Caregivers must take on the responsibility of putting the needs of his or her spouse above their own. This is a HUGE responsibility to bear. However, it is very rewarding.

Within this role, making sure your wife remains on drug therapy is vital. Martha was on Avonex almost two years. Those damn shots get old mighty quickly. We were always surprised to hear the shot compliance statistic at MS talks. Surprisingly, compliance is only about 50% long term for those on shot regimen, according to many physicians. I found that statistic to be staggering.

I know there were numerous times when Martha wanted to just have a normal Friday night without a shot. I told her, "No honey, I know you do not want the shot, but you HAVE to take it." She would always unwillingly oblige and let me stick her. Oh how I hated those long damn needles!

Medication management becomes important when you travel also. The airlines require a letter from your physician authorizing you to carry a needle on an airplane if you are on shot therapy. And then you have to pack it in dry ice for a long voyage or a freezer ice pack for shorter hauls. Even if you are not traveling a long distance by plane or cruise ship, you still have to pack your medication. And for us on Avonex, that always meant adding it to the cooler!

The fourth major role shift, in my opinion, is that of sacrifice and compromise. If you love the outdoors and used to do things together like boating or camping in the summer, those days are over, my friend. These activities must be scheduled differently and tailored to the specific environmental situations.

Martha and I can usually get a nice walk in during the early morning hours before it gets to hot and humid. She still must wear her cooling vest though. We purchased the vest from Polar. And when I still had my little boat, we would go cruising on cool days or in the evenings. Additionally, you will find yourself walking the malls with your wife inside in the air conditioning or going to museums in the summer. You still must plan some fun things, but if heat sensitivity is a factor, adjustments must be made.

Do not give up your hobbies. If you do, this will cause you to resent your wife and that is not a very good idea and will negatively influence your ability to be an exceptional caregiver. You just have to change the "fun" things you do together. Martha and I loved to go to the new mall in downtown Norfolk that was built in 2002, called McArthur Mall. It was a wonderful mall and has movie theatres and a variety of shops.

She loved to go to Harry and David's and get a free sample cup of coffee and then go right outside the store and sit on the comfortable padded bench seat. Then we would watch people for about thirty minutes. It was a blast to watch people interact in public. Typically, on most occasions, we would run into someone we knew.

Another activity we now enjoy together is going to the bookstore, whether at Barnes and Noble at the mall, or the store on Independence Boulevard at Virginia Beach if we were out that way. The most difficult part for me was to plan these "indoor" events on a beautiful sunny day when it was 85 degrees Fahrenheit outside and I wanted to be walking, boating or fishing. In my case though, I am so blessed that my wife Martha is doing so well. I give God thanks each day for this blessing. My heart goes out to those caregivers who must care for their spouse who is not doing very well. It is easy to get depressed when you see your life change and your dreams put on hold. Although her MS is in check for now, our life has changed. We have adapted well to the "new normal" as I mentioned earlier.

Even though Martha has MS, she does not look like she is sick, and most people would never know she has the disease. But coping with this disease does take its toll on her. We have come to simply enjoy the simpler things in life.

Despite your illness, please remember the old adage, "The glass is always half full." This statement rings true in ALL instances, in my opinion. I read a familiar line in another book recently, stating that "Winners never quit and Quitters never win!" This is so true.

I have been working now for thirty years and I can tell you for certainty that how you solve problems and overcome adversity is ninety percent attitude and only ten percent situational. So husbands, if you find yourself overwhelmed and in despair right now, take five and regroup. You have to reprogram your brain. Many years ago, I learned one simple technique but it takes practice. This technique is: "Do not even process negative thoughts! When they start to enter your brain, BLOCK them." You can master this technique but it does take practice.

Chapter 9

SHOT NIGHT

When Martha was first diagnosed, I went with her to Dr. Pellegrino's office where we sat in the waiting room looking at the patient drug kits and pamphlets to decide which drug she would begin taking: Avonex, Rebif, or Copaxone, Looking at the materials, it became evident that she wanted the weekly injection called Avonex. Having any kind of shot is bad enough, so having just one injection per week was the best that we could expect.

Dr. Pellegrino explained the pros and cons of each drug and said it was our decision, since most of these platform drugs work similarly. He stated "if you don't like shots, then maybe the weekly injection is right for you. It is a personal decision but, in your case, I would recommend Avonex." After hearing his opinion on this matter, it was a no-brainer for us.

So we took the packet home and scheduled an in-service with the shot nurse. Without hesitation, Martha placed a call to the nurse on her cell phone during our return home. Our oldest daughter Elizabeth was still at home and she joined us for the in-service. Since she aspired to become a physician or a nurse practitioner, this would be great training for Elizabeth to administer the injection to her mother.

The nurse came to our house a week later and instructed us how to administer the injection. I told Martha I would give her the injections so the nurse trained my daughter Elizabeth and me how to do it. When the nurse opened the package, all our eyes were affixed to the length of the needle; it looked absolutely huge! I thought to myself, "Boy! What a big, long needle!"

My most significant yet basic challenge with shot therapy was how to pop the cap off the syringe, given my little "Jimmy Deans," as Elizabeth called them. She was referring to my chubby fingers, of course! I chew my fingernails, so it was even more difficult to do this. The nurse suggested we inject Martha in her thigh, since the muscles there were larger. She demonstrated to us exactly how to inject her and that is how we planned to administer her first Avonex injection.

The next day, I planned to cook a quiet, savory dinner and attempted to set calm, relaxing mood. We had a few beers and watched a movie on TV. I told Martha around 7 PM, "You better take your Aleve; your shot is in one hour."

She remarked, "Great! I can't wait."

I knew she was anxious about it, as was I. About 7:30 PM, I took the injection out of the refrigerator in order to warm it to room temperature. About thirty minutes later, I gave Martha her first injection in her right thigh. The needle felt bigger than it looked when I plunged it into my wife's thigh.

She exclaimed, "Ouch!" when the needle went in. I literally could feel her pain. I did my best to quickly inject her like throwing a dart, as the nurse had instructed me. It was still scary and everything seemed as if it was in slow motion for a few brief seconds. After the injection, we ate some dinner and soon she went to bed.

As we had been told, later that night, Martha felt like she had the flu. This was the major side effect of this drug. She had sweats and what appeared to be a fever and aches and pains. All she could do was to try and sleep it off and stay hydrated. Oh how we looked forward to our new paradigm of shot night on Friday nights! This was a bitter pill to swallow but we tried to make the best of it. We were in this "MS thing" together.

Being an avid walker before coming down with MS, it quickly became apparent that a shot in the leg was not going to work. Martha remarked how sore her right leg was the next day. We had to cut our two mile walk short by about half a mile that day.

We decided right then and there that we would try injecting the drug in her upper arm the next time, right in the abductor muscle. So, the following week, I iced down the injection site a few minutes prior to the needle stick. I grabbed that big muscle in her upper arm and squeezed it between my fingers and then quickly inserted the needle, again like throwing a dart. Martha winced a bit but this was easier and less painful than getting the shot in her leg. She hated getting these injections and I hated giving them to her, but we had no choice so we had to grin and bear it. We are fortunate to have great health insurance which helps us to afford the drug. Each week, we changed to the next arm. This method worked well and became our weekly routine from that time forward.

My daughter Elizabeth seemed uneasy about administering the injections to Martha so I had to do them all the time. Thirty days after Martha was diagnosed, I was put on a travel assignment by my job for a period of three months. I would travel for two weeks at a time, and then would have a weekend or a few extra days off before traveling to the next site. Needless to say, Martha was not a happy camper when she learned of this work schedule.

During my absence, Elizabeth attempted to inject Martha, but it was too uncomfortable for both of them so Martha decided to go to the doctor's office to have the nurse inject her. She would take the Avonex out of the refrigerator and put it in her purse, take her Aleve, and then off she went for her weekly injection. The traffic on a late Friday afternoon was heavy and it added stress to her day when she had to travel to the doctor's office to get her injection. After the injection, she would come home, relax, eat dinner and go to bed. This worked well during my absence.

Martha always had some interesting stories about the people whom she met at Dr. Pellegrino's office. The humbling aspect of these encounters is that despite her illness, Martha met individuals who were much worse off than she was. I remember her telling me the story of the lady who was having seizures and had just lost her driver's license. At least Martha had her mobility and independence. Furthermore, Martha was still able to work at the school up the street. Yes, it was harder to work now, but at least she had a job.

Martha is a strong lady and a fighter. I believe her fighting attitude and strong faith in God has given her a graceful ability to cope with MS and to make lemonade out of lemons, so to speak. We realized very quickly that she had to come to grips with her changed life, adjust and move on. However, this does not mean you stop living. I remember one comment Dr. Pellegrino made that has stuck with me ever since. He said, "Don't let MS change your personality. Still be who you are and just learn to live within your new limits. You can still have fun; it's not like you have cancer and it is not going to kill you!"

Martha still becomes angry every now and then, but these moments are more fleeting now. She has found her purpose since she retired from her full time job due to disability. She helps others with disabilities and is actively involved with the local MS chapter.

Throughout all these encounters, Martha would encourage these folks and uplift their spirits. She just has a knack for being able to do this. She is such a people's person. She can start a conversation with a stranger at the grocery store checkout counter and make them feel so at ease.

Once I returned to my normal work duty schedule, I resumed giving her the injections and this was much easier on her. I decided right then that I would make shot night even more special. We realized that life would no longer be the same for Martha and she had to cope with this disease as best as she could. And I was her major support system. I delved into my recipes and would start planning a gourmet meal for Friday night earlier in the week. I made sure I had all the fresh ingredients on a Thursday night to make our "dinner date" for Friday since we did not go out much because money was tight. Friday night meals were Chicken Florentine or fresh grilled fish (striper or flounder that I recently caught in the

Chesapeake Bay which is one of the finest fisheries in the whole world).

No matter how rough my week had been, my focus on Fridays is always on my wife and how to make the next few hours extremely enjoyable for her, given that she would have to have her shot by around 8 or 9 PM that night. I tried to keep the conversations light and I doted on her. She was also calm, after having her weekly massage with Tina.

Sometimes, during the summer in that first year, we would go out early, leaving home at 4:30 PM, and walk around the mall a bit and grab a light dinner. We would each get an appetizer, a beer, and split an entrée. We parked at the mall and after dinner on Granby Street we walked back to the mall, got in our car and drove home. We were usually home by 8:30 PM in time for her to get her shot.

But on the nights we stayed home, I enjoyed preparing a delicious gourmet meal, especially when I purchased fresh seafood from Larry at the Norfolk Farm Market. He had a supplier in Louisiana and would fly in fresh shrimp and scallops on Thursday mornings. I would make sautéed scallops and Shrimp Alfredo. The least I could do was to make her shot night as enjoyable as I could.

We soon learned about the combination of certain foods that seemed to minimize her flu-like symptoms. One of these foods was sweet potatoes. Also, we found that having a heavy protein such as chicken or fish along with starch like pasta or sweet potatoes helped her have an easier night.

Over time, Martha's resistance built up a bit, and so she did not get as sick as she did at first. She still hated those shots, however. A key factor in minimizing these symptoms was taking two Aleve one hour prior to the injection. In speaking with other MS patients on Avonex therapy, the flu-like symptoms vary across the continuum; they were minor for some and major for others. All I can say is that these symptoms became tolerable for Martha.

I became quite adept at giving her injections, although there was a time or two where I did "miss." Once, I sort of hit the bone in her arm. She did not like that one at all. I felt terrible.

One eventful shot night occurred on our twentieth wedding anniversary. We planned a weekend getaway at the Hampton Inn on Chincoteague Island on the Eastern Shore of Virginia. It was wonderful to escape for a few days; the dog was boarded at the kennel and the kids were farmed out to spend the weekend with friends.

The day was crazy earlier. Martha had her MRI conducted at Depaul Hospital two days prior to us leaving for our trip. The day we left, she wanted to stop by the hospital to pick up a copy of her MRI. She read the report briefly and we were devastated; 7 new lesions! Dr. Pellegrino had requested that she get a baseline MRI since it was almost a year since her initial diagnosis. He felt this was necessary even though Martha said she felt fine.

You can imagine how upset she was. This was not the news she wanted to hear on her anniversary weekend. The scary part of this news was the realization that her disease was still very active and this meant it was progressing. Avonex was doing its job; but the disease was stronger than the treatment at this juncture. Martha and I were scared.

We had attended an MS conference locally a few months prior and met a phenomenal physician named Virginia Simnad. Dr. Simnad was a practicing neurologist at the MS center in Charlottesville on the University of Virginia Campus. We were rather impressed by her understanding of MS, her clinical trials and her aggressive approach to treating individuals like Martha with very active disease progression. Thus, Martha and I discussed our next option.

We drank a beer in our room that evening, and the infamous shot was slated for later. I came down with horrible 24-hour flu and felt miserable, but I had to think of her and not myself. We went out to dinner at the Village Restaurant a few miles from the hotel. When traveling, we always asked the "locals" where the best seafood restaurant was.

Luckily, we had made reservations the night before so we did not have to wait long. Martha had a shrimp dish and I ordered crab cakes. They were delicious and for dessert, we had homemade apple pie that was absolutely to die for. Overall, our meal was fantastic and reasonably priced, and the atmosphere and service was outstanding. It was a restaurant that I would re-visit.

When we returned to the hotel about 8:30 PM, Martha readied herself for bed and I applied some ice to her injection site. She had taken two Aleve at the restaurant. I dosed her up with Avonex and she bedded down for the night.

I brought my laptop with me. The Hampton Inns always have free wireless internet connection in the room so it was convenient. I conducted some online research. I was scared for my wife. Her MS was progressing and there was no other available drug that we knew of. During my research, I investigated Dr. Simnad's website. She conducted various MS trials in Charlottesville and was known for prescribing various combinations of drugs when one drug alone does not combat the progression of MS.

At that point, I decided that Martha needed a second opinion consult from Dr. Simnad. When she awoke a few hours later, we discussed the situation and she agreed. I fired off a quick email to Dr. Simnad's nurse explaining our situation and requested a consult. When we returned home, Martha called Dr. P and he was very agreeable to a consult so he called her. Our insurance plan was a PPO, so no referral was needed.

Chapter 10

TURNING THE CORNER

On that Monday, when we returned home, Martha called Dr. Simnad's office and spoke with her nurse. She acknowledged receipt of our e-mail and stated that she would speak with Dr. Simnad. The nurse re-iterated that Dr. Simnad would briefly confer with Dr. Pellegrino by telephone in order to confirm details, but that there should be no problem in scheduling the consult visit.

We were able to schedule the appointment for the Wednesday prior to Thanksgiving. We were staying in town for the holiday, so it was just a hop, skip and a jump up the road on I64 for two and a half hours to Dr. Simnad's office, from Norfolk to Charlottesville, Virginia. We left early that morning in time to arrive for an 11 AM appointment.

As we were approaching Richmond via I-295, I realized we were extremely low on gas and tried to remain calm while I looked for an exit with a gas sign. You must be careful on this route since sometimes you must traverse several miles before finding the gas station after exiting. Not all the road signs mark the distance to the station before you exit.

I had traveled this stretch of road many times before. I used to be in sales and was very familiar with which exits not to take, especially if you are very low on gas. Once Martha noticed the gas gauge, however, the "I told you to get gas in Norfolk" and other comments erupted out of her lovely mouth ever so effortlessly. I just replied, "I know, honey, I messed up."

After twenty plus years of marriage, a husband finally learns to admit when he is wrong; pride gets thrown out the door. A peaceful marriage is more important than a bruised ego.

We finally found a Costco and quickly pulled into it and gassed up. We had about a thirty minute window and I had already wasted 10 minutes after we exited since we hit a bit of morning rush hour traffic. I was greatly relieved to have a full tank of gas.

I promised myself years ago that I would never run out of gas in either a car or a boat ever again. I will always remember like yesterday when our young daughters were with us in our little thirteen-foot Boston Whaler boat traversing down the intra-coastal waterway in Chesapeake. Elizabeth was about six years of age and Sarah was four years old. We were having a grand time and I remember as we were approaching the bend nearing Coinjock, NC, Martha asked me, "Are you sure you have enough gas? It looks like we can get some down there a few miles."

Obstinately, I retorted, "Yes, we have enough gas, and we don't need to stop! Let's keep having fun. I know this engine and I know this boat."

Stupid me! We had a six gallon gas tank which lasts a long time in a little boat; however, in this case, I had not adequately compensated for the extra weight of our cooler of food and other supplies.

Wouldn't you know it; within a few minutes, the engine began to sputter. I quickly pumped the gas bulb as fast as I could. It was not remaining hard, so I knew then, that we were in fact out of gas. I said to myself, "Oh shit!"

I looked at Martha, and she looked at me, and I could see her lips pursing and the anger writhing in her countenance. At that moment, the engine just died.

I said a quick silent prayer to myself: "God, please protect my family and give me the wisdom to get out of this situation, Amen."

After I tried to calm Martha down, trying to tune out her deafening angry yells and I TOLD YOU SO's, I began to paddle downstream towards the shore. About a half mile away, I spotted a small dock, which signaled that civilization was nearby. As we were half way there, the two-piece wooden oar came apart, and the lower part dropped in the dismal swamp and began to float away.

Martha had a fit and I burst out at her and said, "Just leave me alone! I will get us out of this situation! Just down there a bit is the dock and I will find some gas! Please, honey, just shut up!" I barked.

We were at a rest area just off route 17 and I quickly darted my eyes to locate a vacation traveler who was towing a boat. My plan was to plead with this individual to give me a few gallons of gas which I would gladly pay for, even double! My six gallon gas tank was empty and it was getting late in the day and I needed to get us back to the boat ramp at Lake Drummond. I found someone in about five or ten minutes. Those few minutes seemed like an hour, though.

He was a young father and had his family with him, so he could understand my plight quite well. I was so obliged. I thanked him, uplifted a quick prayer of thanks to God, and then I ran back to the dock with the full, heavy gas can. As I was approaching the dock, Martha's eyes caught mine and I gave her the thumbs up sign. She was trying to keep the kids calm.

I pumped the gas bulb furiously and quickly. The engine started up immediately. We cast off and away we went, headed for home. It was near dusk at that time and the swamp seemed eerie for us, then.

We arrived at the medical complex for Martha's appointment with Dr. Simnad twenty minutes prior to her scheduled appointment time. I dropped her off in front of the office building so she could hurry in and check in with the receptionist while I parked the car. She was a bit anxious, as we had discussed our options on the trip up. Martha had conducted her own research on this new drug called Antegren, and it looked promising. We looked forward to Dr. Simnad's opinion as to whether or not Martha was a candidate for this new drug therapy.

Martha's appointment lasted about an hour. Dr. Simnad took a very thorough history. I was fortunate to be present for the appointment. Her demeanor was so calming, yet authoritative; it gave you a sense of confidence in her ability to effectively diagnose and treat you as a patient. At the end of her appointment, Dr. Simnad recommended three options for Martha. The first was to begin taking Amantadine, which is a drug prescribed to Parkinson's patients, but it works well to

combat fatigue in MS patients. It stimulates the dopamine receptors in the brain. This was welcome news for Martha. Her daily battles with fatigue were wearing her down. This drug would bring her immediate relief from the fatigue.

The second option she recommended was for Martha to begin infusions of Antegren. "This is a monthly infusion and was just released by the FDA today," she explained.

Dr. Simnad briefly described to us how this drug works to block the T cells from ever entering the brain barrier; thus, if you keep these active cells out of the brain, you effectively stop the progression of MS any further. The thing that excited us most about Antegren was hearing Dr. Simnad explain that this drug was "the most powerful drug available to fight relapsing-remitting MS." The way it worked was to basically stop the demyelination process in the brain from occurring. We were very encouraged by this news since she agreed that Martha's MS was progressing rather rapidly.

The third option for Martha was to schedule a follow-up appointment with one of Dr. Simnad's associates, the neuropsychologist, who would conduct a neurological testing exam in order to provide Martha with a baseline of her cognitive abilities right now. We thanked her for her time and Martha did schedule the follow-up appointment in about a month or two.

When we left the office, we drove up the road about a mile and stopped for lunch at this great little Mexican Restaurant. We ordered two coronas and enjoyed our chips and fajitas. We thanked God for Dr. Simnad and the fact that we had attended the conference in Virginia Beach where we met her. Everything happens for a reason and our "purpose" for going to that MS talk that day was to meet Dr. Simnad.

On the trip home, Martha seemed elated; I could see in her eyes that glimmer of hope that life was going to be OK. She now had this new drug to help fight her MS. Martha whipped out her cell phone and her insurance card and began making the calls to the insurance company to discuss authorization for payment for Antegren. Biogen Idec had also instructed us to call one of their case managers who could intervene with our insurance company to speed up the approval process. At the time, our insurance company was Cigna Healthcare.

Fortunately, Cigna indicated it was aware of this new therapy to treat MS and would cover the infusions. The cost of the monthly infusions (billed to the insurance companies) at that time was several thousand dollars per month. Today, it is even more expensive. Compared to the cost of Avonex, the difference was marginal so it was a no-brainer for us to switch to Tysabri.

Next, Martha called the home infusion company in Norfolk to inform them of her plans to start infusion therapy at their office. Their name was Home Choice Partners. As soon as Martha arrived back home, she stopped by Walgreens to drop off her prescription for Amantadine, which Dr. Simnad had written for her.

Martha and I felt that if we could get her disease under control from this point forward, she could maintain a reasonably good quality of life. She could still function quite well with a few limitations. We knew eventually she would have to retire from full-time work at the school. What she would do and could do next, was still up in the air.

I truly believed that my wife now had a new mission in life; she was determined to get her MS under control with new therapy and to continue to develop her expertise as a patient advocate. We would just take things one step at a time. We praised God for this newfound hope and felt blessed more than ever. We had much to be "thankful" for this Thanksgiving, which was the next day.

We planned a quiet meal at home with just our immediate family that year and we contemplated the recent events and how life might stabilize for Martha.

Chapter 11

BIOGEN IDEC – PATIENT ADVOCACY

Biogen Idec created a Patient Advocate program in 2004 and was in the process of recruiting new advocates when Martha learned of this from Tony Nichols, the local Biogen drug representative whom we befriended at local MS conferences. Tony gave Martha the name of Pamela Raglin, the Coordinator for the program.

I remember when Martha learned about this program. She told me, "That is what I want to do. I love public speaking and, with this program, I can get paid for speaking and help inspire people with MS at the same time."

Martha contacted Pamela and began discussions with her about becoming an advocate. Biogen wanted advocates who were taking Avonex and could speak positively about their experiences at PEP events. A PEP event is a Provider Education Program sponsored by the drug company. These local PEP events usually had a dinner or breakfast program where a physician and a patient advocate spoke. The programs offered a question and answer session at the end.

The patient advocates were asked to speak about their personal experiences for about fifteen to twenty minutes. They were not allowed to render any medical opinions; they were instructed to remind the audience that MS affects everyone differently and that they are just sharing "their story" and would defer any medical question to the physician. The drug company paid the physicians a stipend for their presentation also. This made Martha feel so proud that she could make some extra money, doing what she loves—talking with people and inspiring them!

Martha was accepted into the Patient Advocate Program in January 2005. She had participated in several Biogen Idec conference calls where Advocate Coordinator Pam Raglin instructed them on general guidelines on how to develop an effective Patient Advocate presentation. Martha's mission as a Patient Advocate was to present her story of how MS has affected her and her success with the drugs she is taking. At the time, when she first became an advocate, she was taking Avonex, the weekly infusions of interferon.

Martha was scheduled to present her first Patient Advocate talk in March 2005 in Newport News, VA. She had several months to prepare and practice her presentation. I assisted her with developing a PowerPoint presentation with slides and bullet points and pictures about her story. She had such a great story to tell and my technical knowledge and PowerPoint wizardry made for a winning combination. Before she could present, Biogen Idec required that Martha has her slides approved by them. Furthermore, she had to conduct a mock presentation to Pamela Raglin. Her presentation was fantastic and we continued to polish it. I burned it to a CD and Martha mailed it to Pamela. Her presentation had an overall theme of "Keep Moving." It included pictures of her family, her doing yoga and physical therapy, our team walking in the Fifty-mile Challenge Walk, and was inter-twined with bullet points to convey her message.

Pamela was very impressed and gave Martha the green light. A week before her presentation, I timed her, and gave her honest feedback about her presentation. She was ready and I knew she would knock it out of the ballpark. Her first presentation in Newport News with Dr. Patrick Parcells of Hampton Roads Neurology went smoothly. I was so proud of her and she was poised, positive and promoted enthusiasm in the audience. She moved and inspired the attendees with her story. I knew right then that Martha was making a difference.

Although Martha had received two infusions of Tysabri before her first Advocate talk, she was instructed NOT to mention this, since the drug had just been pulled from the market. The focus of her talk was on Avonex. Avonex was the right drug for her at the time. The problem, though, was that this drug was not quelling the MS enough. She was still having relapses, but working through them. And she was able to briefly tell patients that she had two Tysabri infusions prior to the drug being pulled from the market.

What excited me the most was that in January 2005, Martha was informed of the first ever national Patient Advocate Conference, scheduled for May 2005 in Boston on Mother's Day and it was going to be a huge event. I was able to accompany her on the trip, and we were excited since the agenda included educational programs about new MS drugs and scheduled patient advocate training.

Tysabri had just been recently approved in the US and Europe and infusions were occurring rapidly. This was great news for the drug company. Biogen was excited and was in full swing, promoting the drug. Since the conference was already planned for Spring 2005, there was no way Biogen could cancel it even though the drug was voluntarily pulled from the market in February 2005.

We were so excited about this trip. I wanted to plan something special for Martha on Mothers' Day but I lacked fresh ideas. Now we were anxiously awaiting an all-expense paid trip to Boston! Neither of us had ever been to this wonderful city. The conference began with a reception on Thursday evening, a full day program on Friday with a dinner and a half day program on Saturday. We decided to spend Saturday night on our own and flew back Sunday afternoon.

Flying in to Logan International Airport was one of the coolest flights I have ever taken. I love the water. As you approach the airport, you are flying right over Boston Harbor. We arrived around 10:30 AM and we took a cab to our hotel, the Royal Sonesta, right on the waterfront. The hotel accommodations and scenery were breathtaking.

Martha was tired from traveling and was able to rest in the afternoon so she would have enough energy for the reception. We made the decision that week that she would take her infusion on Wednesday evening so we would not have to mess with traveling with Avonex. She was a little groggy that Thursday morning when we left town in Norfolk but she felt OK and was glad that she did not have to be injected during the trip.

When one has MS and you have to travel by airplane, you are required to have a letter from your physician stating that you have MS, and the drug you are taking must match the drug you have packed in your carryon bag. And, of course, you must have the medication on ice pack, which adds an extra complication. And since 9·11, carrying a syringe on board is a bit more complicated these days. For all of these reasons, we decided it was easier to just take the injection two days earlier that week.

Martha seemed well rested and after both of us took a nice shower, we got dressed for the reception, all the while admiring the beautiful waterfront from our bedroom window. We felt so appreciative to be there to celebrate Mothers' Day, and to meet new people and learn about MS.

My vivid memories of the reception include the gargantuan diver scallops wrapped in bacon, drinking Belgian beer, and being served by waiters in tuxedos. It was outstanding. Beef tenderloin and turkey medallions were also served. They truly were some of the best foods I have ever eaten.

We met some really nice people. I remember one lady whom Martha and I nicknamed "Martini lady." She was walking with the aid of a cane but could still ambulate pretty well. She proceeded to knock back about three martinis and was "feeling no pain!"

We also met a real nice couple from Pennsylvania. Rocky was the husband and he had MS. They were from Philadelphia and he was battling a pretty aggressive strain of RRMS but on Avonex therapy and tolerating it well. He was still working full-time, however. His wife was beautiful and they were the proud parents of two teenage kids.

We learned about the most current treatments for MS and were taught the major aspects of the disease at this conference. The network of MS Patient Advocates we met represented the cream of the crop; these folks were the fighters. They had a disease but each one had an engaging story to tell others about their courageous battles with multiple sclerosis. When individuals share their fears, their struggles and their successes with others, it truly does inspire the audience.

Most of the patient advocates were doing well, but not all of them. I remember "scooter lady." She had recently had her last dose of Novantrone, a major chemotherapy drug. She was having difficulties walking on her own. We assisted her in and out of the van with her scooter when we saw her when we were going on one of our excursions. Despite the gravity of her disease, she still pressed forward with a strong will to beat the disease.

The information we learned at this conference convinced Martha and me that when Tysabri would be re-released, she would resume taking it despite the risk of PML. We knew the risk of contracting PML and, at a risk ratio of 1000 to 1; we both concluded her risk of getting worse was greater than the risk of contracting PML if she did not take the drug. We were told that the drug company was in the process of doing a thorough investigation and we were confident that the drug would be reviewed by the FDA and it would return to the market in the near future.

Break-out sessions for care-givers were scheduled and I really enjoyed them. That gave each of us caregivers the opportunity to learn from each other and we were presented with resources to teach us how to support our loved ones even more. I remember meeting a couple from Newport News, Steve and Lorrie Brantley. She was a retired Air Force Lt. Colonel and she had significant disability with MS. She walked with the aid of a walker. Steve and I got to know each other at the caregiver's session and exchanged e-mails and phone numbers.

During our personal time, Martha and I enjoyed wonderful dining and sight-seeing while in Boston. We had dinner at Legal Seafood one night, which was outstanding. We took a trolley tour of the city, as it was very windy and rainy on our free Saturday afternoon. The tour guide was extremely knowledgeable. We were initially considering taking a Duck Boat tour but later decided against it and chose this one because of the weather. On our own, we took a bus to the local campus of MIT. What a wonderful institution it was! Unfortunately, we didn't have enough time to see Harvard University. That will have to wait until another time.

For a city as large as Boston, Martha and I were impressed with the overall friendliness of the populace. People were extremely polite and helpful in Boston. We both agreed that this was one of our favorite cities and we hoped to return again for another Biogen-sponsored event.

We left for the airport around 2 PM on Sunday since we had a 3:30 PM departing flight. It was very windy and raining for the most part of our trip. I remember my oldest daughter's humorous remark when we found ourselves stuck at the airport on our return journey because our flight was delayed. She said, "Well, it sucks to be you right now!" She is so darn funny. I just love her sense of humor. We were tired but, at the same time, we were happy to have embarked on such a wonderful trip to Boston.

Martha was energized with her advocate training from the recent conference. The local Biogen drug representatives were calling her to schedule her for PEP in Tidewater, Richmond and Williamsburg areas. We fine-tuned her presentation, as she was asked to present about four times annually.

Over the next year, Martha gave two of the best presentations I ever witnessed. My favorite one was the performance she gave in Richmond, Virginia at the Botanical Gardens on a Saturday morning in the early spring of 2006. The attendees numbered about a hundred and she was, again, presenting with Dr. Parcells, her favorite physician presenter. These two had their talk down to a science. They were a smooth and flawless tag team, providers and patient advocates. Martha and I had added some new pictures to this presentation and also reformatted her bullet points. This is, in fact, her finest PowerPoint presentation to date. The audience was highly engaged, as Martha was an exceptional storyteller. One of the themes she learned at the Patient Advocate Conference in Boston was how to give an effective presentation and to drive your overall theme home to the audience. Her theme was "Keep Moving."

So, towards the end of her presentation, with the audience rocking, Martha knew that the next slide was the one that said KEEP MOVING, and before I clicked to the next slide, she asked the audience, "So what does that mean?"

They shouted, "Keep Moving!" and the room shuddered with the renewed enthusiasm of the audience.

She ended her presentation with a loud and appreciative round of applause from the audience.

I told her that was her absolute best presentation ever! Both Tony Nichols and Dr. Parcells concurred. Martha was elated on the drive home. She just kept rehashing the events of the talk and would repeatedly ask me, "So how did I do? What was the best part? Did you like it when I said...?"

I was extremely proud of her. We both agreed, "That presentation was the bomb. Model all the others after that one."

Remember, that part of the challenges as a patient advocate is to keep your presentation fresh, since the physician speakers and the drug representatives can be the same at the next PEP. They do not want to hear the exact same talk again. Martha truly had a knack for giving each successive talk its own flavor, even if she did use some of the same slides. We would try to vary it a bit, adding a new picture here and there.

A situation occurred in the country where one patient advocate presented a slide during a PEP that made a medical claim. The advocates were strictly warned never to do this, but this individual proceeded. Unfortunately, as a result, all the patient advocates in the country were disallowed from having any bullet points in their presentations. They could still have pictures, though.

So Martha and I regrouped and deleted all the slides with bullet points. We added new pictures and changed her storyline a bit. The pictures were more about the elements of her story; staying fit, getting her infusion, me cooking, her practicing yoga, bird-watching, reading, writing notes, etc.

Martha was only one of about thirty Patient Advocates in the country who was taking Tysabri infusions. Locally, in Hampton Roads, she was the primary advocate. Martha had spoken at PEP-sponsored events in North Carolina, Washington, DC, Fairfax, Virginia and Annapolis, Maryland, as well as numerous programs in Hampton Roads. She has continued to perfect her presentations which now include "NO slides." The advocates are no longer allowed to present any audiovisual material; they must just tell their story with no reference materials. To this day, Martha still rocks the audience and the attendees approach her at the end of the evening with congratulatory remarks, being always inspired.

Chapter 12

TYSABRI - THE HOPE THAT LIES AHEAD

Martha was still working full-time at Norfolk Collegiate School, and the stress of working was evident. Having a source for new-found energy with Amantadine certainly helped; however, Martha and I both remembered what Dr. Simnad said. She indicated that Martha had suffered some cognitive dysfunction and more would come. This is a natural progression of the disease.

Slowly but surely, the noises of the school and the job stations that she was asked to work in became increasingly distracting for her, and made it difficult for her to concentrate. She became agitated and would arrive home from work completely exhausted and easily irritated.

Dr. Simnad had discussed with her the option of going out on disability, making it clear to Martha that she would eventually have to face facts and retire from full-time work due to the toll MS was having on her. The everyday stresses Martha was putting on her body with working full-time AND fighting MS started to noticeably affect her mood and energy level.

As mentioned earlier, during the visit to Dr. Simnad, she stated that she thought Martha was an ideal candidate for the newly released infusion therapy, now known as Tysabri. Through the Patient Advocacy program with Biogen Idec, Martha learned that there were quite a few patients around the country who had been taking this new drug during clinical trials for the last two years, and they were doing superbly.

In 2005, Tysabri was not recommended as a first line drug therapy unless patients could not tolerate Avonex or any of the other ABC platform drugs like Rebif, Copaxone or Beta Seron. Clearly, Martha's disease was progressing, so her physician assisted her in getting approval for Tysabri.

Martha and I thoroughly investigated all information we could find about Tysabri and the risk of PML. We did not deliberate too much and both of us quickly agreed that taking Tysabri as a dual therapy was her best option. It was worth the risk in our opinion. We were both anxious and scared at how quickly her MS was progressing.

Martha was able to facilitate approval for her first infusion, effective January 2005. She coordinated her infusion at Home Choice Partners in Norfolk. She knew the owner and had used the company years earlier when she had to have a home infusion of Solumedrol during a relapse. Her physician's practice did not have an infusion center for this new therapy, so Home Choice was it.

I took her to her first infusion. The infusions take one hour and then patients must wait for another hour to ensure no reactions occur. Martha was markedly nervous as they needed to start an IV in her hand or arm. Martha told them emphatically, "Please do not stick my left hand. The veins roll horribly and I cannot bear that pain again."

That is the hand that the infusion nurse stuck during her home infusion of IV Solumedrol when she had a relapse earlier in the year. The pain nearly sent her through the roof.

The infusion nurse was very gentle with Martha and the phlebotomy went well. The IV was started and Martha sat back comfortably in the chair reading a magazine. I was nearby in the patient waiting room. The hour passed by quickly and she did not have any adverse reactions. During the first infusion, I could see the wheels turning in Martha's head about how she was going to make her second infusion a "media event."

Tysabri had just been released by the FDA in November 2005. Martha was extremely excited to be lucky enough to be eligible for the infusion and that our insurance covered most of the cost for this infusion therapy. She and I both felt strongly that this new therapy would keep her disease in check.

Martha loves the media and is quite an MS advocate. She wanted to spread the word of this new treatment option to others in Hampton Roads, so she created a media event in February with two of the local TV stations. Both Channel 10 and 13 News had conducted MS feature interviews with Martha before. A few phone calls later and Martha had the plans with Channel 13 news to cover her second infusion which was scheduled for February 14th, Valentine's Day.

Martha also had a friend from church, Stephanie Harris, who worked for Channel 10 as the medical editor. Martha saw her at church the week before her infusion and mentioned that the competing station was going to be airing the feature segment at the infusion center.

Stephanie excitedly stated that they would like to be included as well.

So on the day of the infusion, it was a zoo as BOTH TV stations' film crews converged at the infusion center. They each put their own twist on the segment. What I liked about my role was having the opportunity to present her with roses during her infusion.

An interview with Martha at the infusion center, a tour of the infusion center to include showing how the drug is prepared, and an interview with her physician, Dr. Thomas Pellegrino, kicked off the feature story for Channel 13. They also filmed Martha getting her infusion and Catherine Barrett, the medical editor for Channel 13, thought it would be a nice touch if I brought Martha flowers since it was Valentine's Day. So, on that particular segment, I came into the room, kissed her, wished her a Happy Valentine's Day and told her I loved her. Then I gave her a dozen roses. Martha was so excited to get home later that day in time to set both VCRs to record each station's news broadcast. Martha enjoys watching herself on TV over and over. Can you blame her? She does a fantastic job!

Very quickly, after the second infusion, Martha appeared to have a new lease on life. She felt great and was confident that MS was not going to take her down the road to disability and disappointment. It seemed like this new drug really makes an impact on people like Martha with relapsing and remitting MS.

Martha and some of the other RRMS patients on Tysabri were on dual therapy, still taking one of the platform injectable therapies. This meant that I was still administering her weekly Avonex injection in addition to her monthly infusions of Tysabri. Both Dr. Pellegrino and Dr. Simnad felt this was the proper course of action, given the quick progression of her disease as indicated by the recent MRI.

Nationally, with the increased publicity of stories like Martha's, MS patients now had another treatment option. Therefore, Biogen Idec increased patient advocacy activities to improve sales, and to offer an improved treatment option that the FDA had determined to be twice as effective as any other drug therapy option for relapsing-remitting multiple sclerosis. Martha was glad that she would be called by the drug representatives in the area to speak at local PEP functions.

February 28th, 2005 was a day we all remember in the MS Community. That is the day that Biogen Idec announced it was voluntarily pulling Tysabri off the market. Three patients had been diagnosed with PML and died. The company thought it was in the best interests of the patient population to pull the drug and have it reviewed for safety.

This news spread rapidly. Martha was very upset. She had just had two infusions and was feeling wonderful and had her hopes back for the first time in a while. What a disappointment this news was! Life, however, needed to be preserved and the risk of PML seemed closer to home with this announcement.

Over the next several months, Martha scoured the internet for any available information on Tysabri and PML and the current status of her "wonder drug." She was anxious since she had to endure several months with no treatment at all. We both began to wonder if the drug would ever return to market, given the current situation.

Through her internet research, Martha stumbled upon a group of MS patients who had been taking Tysabri for years, many who were participants in clinical trials. A lot of these patients had disease much worse than Martha. These patients belonged to an advocacy group called "Patients for Choice." The group was led by David Kaplan. Martha joined this group and they kept in constant communication with each other through a list serve distribution list.

This group's members ranged from patients in California, Idaho, Illinois, Puerto Rico, Virginia, Maryland, and other states, just to name a few. The group had about thirty members. The primary objective of this group was to stay informed about Tysabri's status with Biogen and the FDA. For Martha and many of these patients, Tysabri was the ONLY drug that effectively treated their MS. Many of these individuals were already out on disability, but the motto for the group was that their "choices" entitled them to make the best decisions for their treatment to maintain a quality of life. Most of them had progressive MS or even severe relapsing-remitting MS. Martha and I felt blessed compared to them since she was doing much better than they were.

MS is one of those diseases that when properly treated allows the patient to maintain a certain quality of life. Martha and I did not have many experiences when her disease was stable. Right when we thought we had it fixed and she'd had two Tysabri infusions, the drug was pulled off the market! Needless to say, both of us longed for the opportunity for her to have the choice to take Tysabri again.

The group members began to correspond on issues affecting each other and friendships were made over the internet. Around December 2005, David Kaplan informed the members that an FDA Advisory Panel was going to be held in Maryland in early March 2006. He e-mailed each member the name of the head of this panel so they could write a letter to him requesting to be one of forty-eight patients who were allowed to give a three-minute testimony for or against Tysabri.

I assisted Martha in writing her letter to the physician, asking to be included in the patient testimony proceedings. The deadline was in late January. Martha was notified that she would be allowed to present her testimony to the advisory panel. She was also one of about eighteen members of the Patients for Choice group who were invited to testify in front of the FDA Advisory Panel. All Tysabri patients were instructed to present their views on why Tysabri was a safe and effective drug and why it should be re-released to the market. Each person would have only three minutes for their testimony. This was a very big deal and David Kaplan's advocacy efforts to make this happen were tremendous.

David kept all the members informed about Biogen Idec's investigative efforts surrounding the PML cases. At that time, there were about 3,500 patients who were taking Tysabri. Medical records were reviewed on all clinical trial patients and safety measures were being put into place to monitor patients' health. According to David

Kaplan, Biogen Idec was confident that their due diligent efforts and plan for the re-release of Tysabri would be accepted by the FDA Advisory Panel.

Martha wrote her speech and I edited it. It is challenging to write a concise paper, let alone a concise speech in three minutes which conveys the last two years of one's struggles with MS. Martha worked very diligently on her speech. She practiced it numerous times, as each patient would only be allowed three minutes. The time was very tight. We were forced to write and rewrite, cutting out words and adding new phrases that stated her point more succinctly. Finally, after a few more practice sessions, we were right at two minutes 45 seconds. We were confident in her story

Chapter 13

MAKING HISTORY – FDA TESTIMONY

The date of the Advisory Panel meeting was March 6, 2006. The hearings were being held at the Holiday Inn at Gaithersburg, Maryland, and that is where we had our hotel room. Martha and I left the afternoon of March 5 around noon and drove to Gaithersburg. Traffic was light. Martha was anxious but she practiced her speech a few times on the ride up, so she was well-prepared. I told her how proud I was that she was doing this.

We were close to our destination when my daughter called. I answered my cell phone and could hear her, but when I spoke she could not hear me. This was frustrating. I called her back, and the results were the same. Martha only had one bar of power left on her cell phone. This was not good. I felt uncomfortable being out of town and not being able to be "connected" to my daughters by cell phone.

I had no way to communicate with my daughters. Martha forgot her cell phone charger and only had limited power left. It was during this trip that I figured out how to text message. I was able to text my daughter and hoped I could receive text messages also. Right then, Elizabeth sent me a text message. Voila! I was able to send and receive text messages, and that became our method for communicating. My nervousness was quelled for the time being, knowing that I now had a way to check on my two daughters who were at home alone with our dog Belle.

When we arrived around 3:30 PM and checked in, Martha and I met one of the couples, Mike and his wife Susan, whom we had been corresponding with via email for months prior to that time. It was nice to finally place a face to a name, so to speak. They were a warm, friendly and genuine couple. Mike, however, walked with a cane. His MS was progressing and he recently had suffered a relapse.

Later that afternoon, before dinner, I remembered seeing Mike who was walking with a cane pacing back and forth near the business office. He looked frantic and was upset. I spoke with him and he said he was having difficulty printing his speech. The computer in the business office was not recognizing his thumb drive. I did not have my laptop with me so I tried to assist him by finding a manager and letting him try his thumb drive in another computer.

Trust "Media Martha" to draw an Irish reporter's attention to herself. The reporter was there to report on the events since Elan Pharmaceuticals was the only other drug company in Europe who produced Tysabri for Biogen Idec. I turned around and there was my wife conducting an interview for an Irish TV News Station on the events at hand. Martha loves the camera and she granted the reporter an excellent three-minute interview on the hearing scheduled for tomorrow and her part in this historic event.

The plan was for everyone to meet for dinner at around 6 PM. The people we met who were involved with this advocacy group were varied and phenomenal. The ones who stood out, to name a few, were Cheryl Bloom, ex-pilot from Chicago, and Mike whom we met earlier and was a nuclear engineer. All of these people had their own remarkable stories about how they battled MS.

One couple we met did not have MS but were involved with the group for the cause. They were from Wisconsin. We sat next to them at dinner. They were so kind. I remember telling her that Martha was tired and wanted to go to bed early and because of that we were going to forgo dessert. Nancy had said that she would be glad to bring our dessert to our room later. She said it was cheesecake, so we took her up on her offer. Around 7:45 PM, there was a knock on the door and there was Nancy with our cheesecake. It was delicious. We ate it and savored every morsel. I checked on the girls one last time via text messaging and once I learnt they were all fine, we went to bed around 9:30 PM.

Neither of us slept very well that evening. We were used to a king-sized bed back at home but we were sleeping in a full size bed that night. We were also very anxious about the hearing and Martha's testimony. This hearing was emotionally draining, knowing how important each person's testimony was to the final outcome of Tysabri being re-approved for market release.

The next morning was chaotic! Martha had to check in and obtain her "number" for her testimony. She was number thirty-two out of forty-eight, so she had hours to wait before her turn. There were twelve members on the advisory panel, encompassing a varied skill level from physicians to hospital administrators, and so on. Not

125

everyone who testified at this advisory panel was for Tysabri. One man, who was first to testify, was strongly against Tysabri. His wife was one of the three patients who had recently been diagnosed with PML and then died. His testimony was moving and compassionate. It is difficult to lose a loved one with a disease, due to drug interactions. Martha and I personally had to filter his remarks; we were certainly sorry for his loss, however, we still felt the risk of contracting PML was worth it and wanted Tysabri back on the market. One important thing stuck in our minds during these hearings. The three people who were taking Tysabri and died from PML had compromised immune systems. Our exposure to physician advocacy presentations where we always learned new information during the question and answer sessions had taught us that, in most cases, the person contracting PML already had a compromised immune system and the PML was not completely attributable to Tysabri alone.

The room was rather tense, as emotions were running high. Not all testimonies were personal. Some individuals sent in a videotaped testimony, as they were unable to be physically present. Most of the stories were similar. Even people with primary and secondary progressive MS who were taking Tysabri improved in their motor and cognitive functions. This was encouraging since Tysabri was primarily prescribed for relapsing remitting MS only.

A few hours into the testimonies and there was not a dry eye in the place. We witnessed individuals entering the room on walkers, in wheelchairs, on crutches, in scooters, and walking with a cane. Some participants were so debilitated and exhausted that they had to rest up in their room until just a few minutes before it was time for their testimony. It was easy to estimate one's time for his or her testimony, since each person was only granted three minutes each.

The moderator would let the individual presenting know exactly when their time started. At the end of three minutes, the volume to the microphone was turned off. If the person continued to talk past their allotted three minutes, they could not be heard. The panel was reminded to not accept any additional testimony they may have heard after the microphone was off. There were reporters there from the AP wire, and other groups were videotaping the entire panel hearing.

I remember one couple in particular. He was a physician from Harvard and, at the last minute, he had to testify for his wife. She was still up in the bed and physically unable to get dressed and appear in person. The committee made an exception and let her husband read her testimony in the first person.

The majority of participants gave compelling testimonies as to why Tysabri should be re-released to the market. Martha and I remember one physician who was a neurologist and had MS for years. He stated, "I need this drug to treat myself first, so I can then treat my patients. Without it, I cannot practice medicine."

There was a staging area up on the front row where they seated the next participant. This was much like the on deck person getting ready to bat when the current batter is up at the plate. It was now time for Martha to be "on deck" as she was the next one to testify. It was early afternoon.

She was wearing her pretty blue blouse and black pants and looked confident and poised. I said a quick, silent prayer, asking God to help her with her testimony and to enable her to maintain her composure and also to finish her speech on time. Here is her testimony she presented to the FDA Advisory Panel that day:
****

Why Tysabri Should Be Re-Released

Distinguished Advisory Drug Committee Members:

Thank you for the opportunity to testify before you today. I hope to leave a profound impression on you by the end of my three minutes as I tell you why I think Tysabri should be re-released. My name is Martha Rogers. I am fifty-two years old, a wife, mother of two teenage daughters, and a teacher working thirty hours a week. And I have MS. My "world" as I knew it changed two years ago when I was initially diagnosed with having this debilitating disease. I was happy, working full-time and getting into shape and looking great. Everyday was a joy to live and I was thankful.

I was diagnosed in February 2004 after an attack of optic neuritis which the doctor first thought was a brain tumor. An MRI showed my condition to be Multiple Sclerosis. My neurologist allowed me to choose Avonex since I felt that was the best disease-altering drug for me at the time. I was encouraged by the news about the future release of Natalizumab (Nat-a-liz-uh-mab). My first relapse occurred during the spring of 2004.

128

I was one of the very first patients in Norfolk, Virginia to receive an infusion of Tysabri in January 2005. I was so excited about going on the drug that I was able to get on two local TV stations for the five o'clock news. Channel 10 and Channel 13 news stations aired medical feature stories about this wonderful drug. I received two infusions before Biogen Idec voluntarily withdrew the drug from the market. I felt fantastic within twenty-four hours of my infusion, and could really feel the drug stopping the virus from entering into my brain. I knew that I could face any obstacle with this disease, as long as I had my Tysabri! My fatigue went away and I felt steadier on my feet.

When the drug was withdrawn from the market, Channel 10 News convened a follow-up feature news story on me again, to get my opinions on the impact this withdrawal had for me and many MS patients.

Since February 2005, after the drug was pulled from the market, my MS continues to progress, and I have had two more relapses. Since going off Tysabri and back to Avonex, my symptoms have returned. I received steroid therapy at that time.

I have had to adjust my life in many ways in order to manage the various symptoms of this devastating and unpredictable disease. My particular symptoms include balance and gait issues, constant fatigue, memory and concentration problems, and impaired vision. I have also had to cut back on my hours at work, causing my family financial hardship. The unfortunate aspect of this disease is that it takes effort everyday to be happy; to be thankful about something. The progression of my disease has consumed my thoughts, challenging me to overcome my anger about having MS, and, sometimes, I feel very hopeless, especially when I am in the midst of a relapse.

I urge you to consider the results of the clinical trials to date. These trials have proven that Tysabri has a profound ability to stop the virus from entering the blood-brain barrier. I believe this drug WILL prevent my disease from getting any worse. It is all about maintaining a quality of life. I believe Tysabri is THE BEST DRUG available today for people like me who want to have the "choice" to treat their MS effectively. To date, I believe that no other drug can do what Tysabri can do for people with relapsing-remitting MS.

I urge you to reinstate Tysabri, given the favorable outcomes that I experienced. Do not delay this wonderful treatment option for me and the other 400,000 plus people in the United States diagnosed with Multiple Sclerosis.

THANK YOU!

****

I was so proud of her. Her microphone did turn off even though she went over her allotted time by a few seconds. But she did get most of the way through her testimony. Her story, like most of all of the ones we heard, was so moving and had the familiar theme to it. Martha and these patients simply could not live a quality life with MS if they were unable to choose to take Tysabri. NOT having this drug on the market was not a viable option for them.

What made Martha's speech so believable was the fact that in the year since Tysabri was pulled from the market and she was back on Avonex, her disease had progressed again and she had another relapse. This time; however, she was able to take oral prednisone steroids. But the fact remained; without Tysabri, Martha's condition would continue to worsen, and long-term disability stared her down in the face now more than ever.

As a group, we were confident that our message was heard by the panel and that they would rule in our favor. Later that day, after all the testimonies had been presented, David Kaplan explained that the rumor was "the panel was extremely moved by patients' testimonies and would most likely vote in favor of re-releasing Tysabri, given certain conditions."

David informed us that he would e-mail us all the latest information. It was four o'clock in the afternoon and we needed to leave immediately if we wanted to avoid the traffic on the way home. We said goodbye to all our new friends and wished each other well and congratulated everyone for a job well done. ALL of us were exhausted from the emotional two days that surrounded this historic event.

Once we were safely past the traffic snarls of Washington, DC, I said to Martha, "Let's stop somewhere and get something to eat; it has to be a place where I can get a beer. I need a beer badly. Think about it; we just made history!"

"We need to celebrate our cause," I reasoned, as my mouth was parched.

Chapter 14

SOCIAL SECURITY & DISABILITY

That Christmas, she and I discussed and decided that in the beginning of fall, she would go out on disability. Luckily, she had been paying into a long-term disability plan at work. We were overjoyed that she had the option of getting paid sixty percent of her salary.

The school insurance plan was with Anthem, and their agent for the disability plan was named Allsup. Allsup had an incentive to help Martha apply for disability with the Social Security administration. Once she started to receive payments from social security, their monthly obligations were reduced to fifty dollars. They helped her immensely and told her it would take, at least, a year before getting approved and that, at least, one appeal would be required.

Martha and I had discussed at length the financial impact of her going out on disability and we both agreed that we could handle it and, moreover, it would only be for about a year or so, with a forty percent reduction in income. Remember, when you go out on disability, you receive sixty percent of your income until age sixty-five.

Her health was paramount and, as I mentioned earlier, full-time work was really taking its toll on Martha. Her exhaustion and agitation after a day of work was significant. She deserved some element of happiness and her life had become a "working hell." And I was on the other end of that stick, "getting a licking." So, yes, I must admit that I had a slight self-interest in seeing her retire from full-time work. If she was happier, I would be, too. Remember; "a happy wife means a happy life!"

Martha decided on a Monday morning after soulful deliberation during the weekend that she would quit and go out on disability. She called Will King, the headmaster of Norfolk Collegiate School, but he was not in his office, so she left him a voicemail indicating that she had decided to retire on disability.

Mr. King returned Martha's phone call and it was a cordial one. He told her that he understood and would be glad to help in any way. Thus, the paperwork was initiated and she never returned to Norfolk Collegiate. We had many memories of the school since both our children attended for nine years each, but it was time to move on.

Those next few weeks were busy, with Martha communicating with Allsup. They calculated that Martha would receive $850 per month disability payment. During this time, they would also assist her with the claim to Social Security. They clearly stated; however, that it would most likely be a year and a half before her claim would be settled. "This was typical," we were told.

Being the business major, I dutifully pulled out the budget worksheet and re-analyzed our discretionary expenses to determine what ways we could cut back expenses. The biggest areas that presented plausible opportunities for savings were the following: gifts, dining out, coffees at Starbucks, and clothing expenses for Martha. They were also those cash expenses that she never really tracked before, but that were, now, very important to control.

After carefully choosing my words, I began our discussions on finding yet another new, normal life for Martha out on disability with reduced household income. I explained to her that we could easily live comfortably once she was receiving full disability payment from Social Security but, during this inter-rim period, our lives would be challenging.

She tended to feel a bit "guilty" about not making enough money to support our lifestyle, but I assured her that we could do this together. I stated that she would have to be mindful of her cash expenditures and cut back on some "nice to have's" and focus on the "got to have's." I reminded her that she now had the time to focus on taking yoga classes more than once per week and that was an additional expense. She would have to cut back on gift-giving and coffees at Starbucks in order to have the money for the classes. Yoga was important for her health. A quick little analogy brought to light how those three-dollar coffees at Starbucks can add up; two coffees per week $\mathbf{x}$ 52 weeks $\mathbf{x}$ 5 years = $1560. That is the cost of a nice little vacation for a few days!

Martha was enjoying both her yoga classes and eagerly awaited the classes each week. Some weeks, she attended class twice. She learned moves that she could do at home on her own yoga mat. I am convinced that better fitness aids one in combating the effects of MS on a daily basis. You need both a sound mind AND a sound body.

I think the hardest thing about maintaining a fitness routine is the time constraints. You basically have to tell yourself that you have an "appointment with your body and mind" everyday at a scheduled time, whether morning or evening. I prefer morning, since it raises your metabolism for the whole day and it is a lot easier to fit into your schedule. You have more energy in the morning, anyway. Dr. Oz states that there is a chemical reaction in the brain when you exercise 30 minutes or more, whether it be jogging or walking. This chemical reaction is like a "reset" button for your brain. It literally clears the head of today's issues and lets you focus on the "now." I find that once I dedicate the time to exercise consistently, my body craves it even more!

About nine months elapsed before Martha received a response from the Social Security Administration, via Allsup, that her claim has been denied. This was no surprise. The Allsup representative told us this was standard practice. An appeal process was initiated and we expected that to take at least six months before any action would occur. The unfortunate aspect of this component of our healthcare system is that many people already out of work on disability do not have long-term disability plans to "tide them over" for this one to two years period while their claim is tied up at Social Security administration.

Patients still must continue their drug therapy. Without a working spouse, paying for MS drug therapy alone can put you in financial hardship very quickly. We were fortunate that I have great health insurance with my job. Thankfully, we could still handle our portion of the drug cost plus the co pay which altogether approached $300 per month.

Biogen Idec has a "drug assistance" program for those who do not have insurance. Not having insurance is not reason enough to stop your drug therapy. They can underwrite most of the drug expenses for you. They take their cases on an individual basis, so call your local Biogen drug representative and he or she can assist you.

The phone call came from Allsup, finally, that the last step in Martha's claim process was for her to meet with a psychiatrist for him to evaluate her disability claim and her fitness/ability to work or not to work. When she told me the name of the physician and his office location, I told her I did not recognize the name or the location and that she would have to get directions.

It was an unusually hot day on the day of her appointment and she was running behind schedule. Luckily, Martha had her cell phone with her and was able to call the office for final directions when she was close. She was a bit agitated. At one point, Martha even considered canceling her appointment because she thought she was going to be so late and was lost. Eventually, the receptionist calmed Martha down enough for her to find her way.

Needless to say, when Martha met the physician, she was aggravated, anxious, tired and grumpy. It did not take the doctor long to diagnose Martha as "unfit" for full-time work. Hooray! The appeal process was finally over. Within one week of her visit to this doctor, she had a phone call from the local social security office instructing her to schedule an appointment to conclude her disability claim and to start receiving monthly payments PLUS a lump sum settlement for months she had been out already.

I gladly went with her. At first, I thought I knew where the Social Security Administration was. We headed out into Airport Industrial Park over by Robin Hood Road area. After a quick drive through a few streets, I realized I was lost and had to admit I did not know where the office was. And our appointment was in twenty minutes. Martha's anger stiffened and she gave me a stern look and a quick but loud shrill, "I told you so."

Thank goodness for cell phones! It took me a while to get through but someone finally answered and told me where it was. It was located near Target and Home Depot off Military Highway. I drove as fast as I could. We pulled into a handicap parking spot, jumped out and arrived to pull a number to be seen for our appointment. That whole process seemed a bit silly but then, it is a Federal Government agency!

After about an hour, the lady called our number back and we were promptly seen. She indicated that Martha's claim was all in order and asked us a few questions in order to complete the process. The interviewer informed us that Martha would be receiving a lump sum check for all her monthly payments due since she had been out on disability over a year and a half ago! This amounted to about $8500.00. However, we had to pay back Allsup the amount they paid her during this time, and so we still had those amounts to figure in. The monthly difference in income was around an additional $425 per month from Social Security. So we still grossed well. The other aspect of this process I found quite interesting was that since our youngest daughter, Sarah, was still living at home and under the age of eighteen, she was eligible to apply for social security disability until she graduated from high school. I am so glad I discontinued worrying about how to pay for college a few years prior. This was awesome! Sarah would have around $15,000 that she could put in her 529 school fund. I told her that we needed to protect the principal because the market was tanking back then and we could invest it all in a Certificate of Deposit for one year, since she would not need those monies until then anyway. Off to Wachovia we went and accomplished this. After one year, we opened a money market 529 B plan fund to further minimize risk and earn a marginal return.

Chapter 15

LIQUID GOLD

Martha was working part-time at EVMS as a Standardized Patient. A Standardized Patient refers to the individual assigned a "diagnosis," where he or she must learn the case's history in order to assist the medical students and physician's assistants in their patient encounter training. Students must take a history of the patient in order to determine the correct diagnosis. The Standardized Patient must be careful not to "give up too much information, and to make the medical students work for it to conduct an accurate differential diagnosis."

The Standardized Patient evaluates the student in various areas and provides them with valuable feedback at the conclusion of the encounter. Martha was an outstanding Standardized Patient and was admired by all.

She was fielding calls from the Biogen Idec drug representatives to speak at a patient advocate program every so often so that she could stay busy. Needless to say, she was not very happy about having to take weekly Avonex injections again. But what else are you going to do? That was the strongest drug for her at that time until Tysabri was re-released to the market.

Two years into her battle with MS, Dr. Pellegrino left his neurology practice to become Dean of Eastern Virginia Medical School. Although this loss of her neurologist upset Martha, the plan had already been under consideration. She had been speaking at Patient Education Programs (PEP) with Dr. Patrick Parcells, an MS Specialist in Newport News. He became Martha's new neurologist. The funny thing is that both Dr. Pellegrino and Dr. Parcells completed their residencies together at Yale University and it was Dr. Pellegrino who encouraged Dr. Parcells to move to Tidewater years ago. It is a small world!

The news came on June 5, 2006 that the FDA had approved Tysabri for re-release as monotherapy as early as July 2006. Martha quickly contacted her infusion center to schedule her next infusion. We both sighed deeply, grateful that this drug was now going to be available again. It was the only drug we felt was safe for Martha to take that was capable of arresting the further progression of her MS.

Dr. Parcells instructed Martha to cease the Avonex injections for thirty days prior to the Tysabri infusion. She didn't mind this even though she had just had a relapse a few months prior. We both were confident that life would be more manageable once she was on Tysabri again.

The last eighteen months had been long, with Tysabri being withdrawn from the market. Martha was constantly plugged into the latest updates on Tysabri so she knew exactly when it would be available at her doctor's infusion center. As soon as it was available, she called the office and was informed that she could restart her monthly infusions beginning August. This news elated Martha and she regained a bit of confidence and hope.

Her monthly infusions continued to be an enjoyable event. Yes, I said "enjoyable." Martha convinced herself to make the infusion a pleasurable experience since she has to have the drug to live the quality of life she wants and needs, so why not enjoy it? Martha is a motivator. Her infusion nurse, Kim, loves her and all the new patients she meets adore her. Martha is one of those individuals who just "lights up the room" when she enters. She has a unique way of making people feel special and the moments they share are memories for a lifetime. After her infusion, she would drop by the Trader Joe's store nearby and purchase a few specialty items like their Mandarin Orange Chicken. They continually had food and coffee samples showcasing new foods and coffees available.

It was evident that the drug Tysabri was carrying out its purpose. Once Martha was on the drug again, she had just a minor disease progression but NO more relapses. It was time for her to regain her normal life again.

Once Tysabri was back in full release, Biogen Idec began to call Martha again to speak at local Provider Education Programs. Martha would call me on the cell phone and excitedly restate the venue for her next program. She loved making extra money from being a motivational speaker, and, more importantly, she inspired dozens of folks with MS at these talks. Her story is so moving and engaging that everyone in the audience can relate to it and to her. I attended these programs with her whenever possible. It is truly inspiring to witness her deliver what she has practiced and refined for the last five years. My favorite part is always how she conveys her

MS diagnosis. She builds up the story, pulling in the audience each minute as the story unfolds. The fact that she and her ophthalmologist, Dr. Kerner, thought she had a brain tumor is remarkable, since it was such a scary proposition for one to embrace. So when she tells the audience, "When my doctor came into the exam room 'smiling', I felt relieved since I thought to myself that she couldn't be smiling if I had a brain tumor."

My other cherished memories of her advocate talks are towards the end of her program when she emphatically states, "So, since I have been on Tysabri, I have had 'zero' relapses, and 'zero' new disease activity," gesturing with her fingers and drawing a big "0" in the air.

She always concludes by encouraging the audience to "Do your part, since the drug is doing its part. Stay motivated, stay involved, stay physically and mentally fit, and 'keep on moving.'"

I have often remarked to Martha that her gift of telling her story to others with MS is founded on the principle that if just one person decides to start taking Tysabri and he or she is not doing well, it is a life changer. She does make a difference in each talk she gives.

As I have stated earlier, it is all about the quality of life one lives. In this day and age, you surely do not know what is around the corner, so make the most of each and everyday. My motto has always been 'Carpe Diem,' which means, "Seize the Day."

Martha's gig at the medical school required her to work more often and she relished the fact that she now had energy to work half to full days on occasion. It was difficult for her to work even a half day, especially if it was in the afternoon; morning hours are best for her. It was critical for Martha to rest up before a big day of work to reserve her energy.

More often than not, Martha would "overbook" her schedule by accepting cases with EVMS as a standardized patient when those dates were side by side with other key events. She created her own stress by doing this; however, she longed to stay busy and absolutely loved making extra money. Her response to me was invariably the same:

"We need the money, so I am going to do it!"

She was correct. We always DID need the extra money.

For whatever reason, in our married life, we have never had that financial cushion to allow life "ease up on us a bit." It seems as though there is always another emergency around the corner!

As Martha begins her morning tea-sipping in bed, she often pulls her little pocket calendar out of her purse, and review her schedule for that week and the upcoming week. It truly imparts a feeling of accomplishment and success that she is employed part-time and has work scheduled on a regular basis. I like to tease her by remarking:

"Honey, you get paid to push the pillow whether you work at EVMS or not. That is a pretty good deal, with your Social Security disability income."

But thank God we have this income! Martha achieved success with her third and final trip to the Social Security

Administration in 2010 when she received Medicare part B insurance. But this task was not easy. She ended up waiting a lot of time and having "this" form filled out, only to be told that, in addition, she needed "that" form as well. So she had to go obtain additional information and then return.

The second time she returned to the office, the lady at the front counter greeted her in a very unfriendly manner and made her visit untenable. She returned home exasperated, and remarked, "I am never going back to that damn office!"

I said to her, "Honey, you have to go back. We are almost at the finish line. I would do it for you if I could, but YOU have to complete this. I will get you the information you need and fill out the forms for you. All you have to do is to sign them."

The additional information they required was proof of coverage from my prior employer, Northrop Grumman. They had to show continuity of coverage for her with that insurance as primary during the period of her MS diagnosis. So, armed with the final bits of required information, we held our breath and I said goodbye. I remember telling her, "Good luck, honey, you are finally there. There is no way they CANNOT grant you insurance now. This is all they told you that you needed to supply to them in order to process your part B application."

About two weeks later, her Medicare part B card arrived in the mail. We were truly ecstatic, since we knew this additional coverage would save us, at least, five hundred dollars per month.

When she was first diagnosed, we did not understand how much Medicare would pay towards her Tysabri infusions as secondary insurance. Because of the size of my company, Medicare is her secondary insurance. She is covered as a dependent on my insurance policy which is primary. So, now, most of her medical expenses are for medical office visit co pays and prescription drug co pays. Her Medicare Part B premium is $135 each month, and is deducted directly from her disability check. This is money well spent.

We were extremely thankful that she was on her Tysabri regimen once again. Her liquid gold regimen could be resumed again. By "liquid gold", I mean that this drug is as precious and highly valuable because without it, Martha wouldn't be the same person that she is today. Neither would I.

From a spouse/caregiver perspective, it is not easy living with MS, as I like to remind Martha. She lives with "having" the disease. I live with "her coping with the disease." Thus, I like to state that I live with it since it has impacted our marital relationship in many ways. Yes, she has been deprived of favorite activities like going to the beach, and boating and hiking in the summer months because of the heat. And I have been deprived of them as well because we both used to enjoy those activities together. The most difficult aspect of MS that I loathe is how it simply "sucks" the energy out of Martha. She has to make adjustments and spend a lot of time resting in her bed, reading books, watching TV and yakking with her family and friends over the telephone.

Chapter 16

STAYING FIT

A healthy body starts with a healthy mind and a determination to stay focused on the objective. For Martha, that objective was beating MS by not letting it rob her of a decent quality of life. As mentioned in earlier chapters, Martha and I were both relatively fit.

Not only is Martha strong-willed; she is strong physically. Her consistent walking and yoga have kept her fit for years. Martha was always a fast walker even before MS. I remember, before my walking days began in earnest, that I had difficulty in keeping up with her. I was overweight at the time and didn't exercise regularly. But in a weird kind of way, her diagnosis of this unpredictable disease in 2004 caused us to re-evaluate our health priorities. It was extremely important for her to stay as strong as she could, in order to fight the early onset as effectively as possible.

During the early years of MS, Martha was on weekly Avonex shots as her frontline drug therapy. Again, let me re-iterate one significant point made by the physicians at all the MS patient advocate programs:

"Get on drug therapy treatment immediately upon diagnosis of MS."

Martha was able to continue her walking with her friends, although adjustments had to be made due to her reaction to heat. She would meet her friends early in the morning before work in order to beat the heat and get in a quick two to three miles walk.

Early on, her balance was quite off. I recall telling our Eucharistic Minister at church that we could not carry up the gifts when asked because since Martha was unsteady on her feet. She had to hold onto my arm when approaching the altar to receive Eucharist. Her first mission afterwards was to find a reputable physical therapist close to our house, so it would be convenient for her to attend regular physical therapy sessions.

Martha found a practice called North Shore Sports and Physical Therapy up at Wards Corner, within two miles of our house. Her therapist was named Lisa Koperna. Lisa was wonderful and her techniques produced immediate results with Martha. She strengthened her legs and helped her regain her balance. Martha regained her steadiness and gait by "balancing" on what I called the "wobble/weeble ball." This contraption was a small board placed on top of the ball and her goal was to rock from side to side while maintaining her balance.

Over time, she mastered this routine and regained her confidence and composure. During the period, from 2004 to 2008, with the patient advocate programs when Biogen Idec still allowed the advocates to use slides in their presentations, I remember the pictures of her that we shared with the audience on the "Strength" section of her speech. There was a picture of her balancing on the wobble/weeble board.

Therapeutic yoga emblazoned Martha with calmness and kept her muscles limber. She attended yoga classes in Ghent twice a week. I know, for a fact, that her physical activities with other women kept her going. The actual physical activity itself was truly beneficial; however, the social aspect of her workouts aided her greatly and helped her stave off depression. Depression is so common a side effect of MS and its drugs that it is important to avoid solitude which only promotes further depression. And Martha certainly does have the gift of gab. One time when I was at a Medical Group Management Conference, the speaker was discussing communications in the session. What he told us made perfect sense to me. He said that women "talk for the love and joy of talking," and that men "talk to solve problems." I found that to be both fascinating and true. And I can confidently state that his premise holds true for Martha and me. She loves to give me the blow by blow details, and all I want to know is the bottom line.

So there I was, Mr. Couch Potato, drinking my beer and watching sports, and then WHAM! My wife is diagnosed with MS. Well, I told myself then, "Dude, you better get your act together because this is an unpredictable disease and you need to be healthy so you can take care of her." I must admit I was scared initially about the long-term prospects for her life with MS, but then I convinced myself to focus on only those things within my own control. And first and foremost was my health. I had to stay healthy so I could take good care of her. Thus began my diet and exercise regimen. I was never really interested in joining a gym for exercise. I was content with my walking and home calisthenics. I also liked to play golf and to fish.

Martha and I decided that we would get involved with the MS community, form a walking team, raise money for the society, and get in shape at the same time. That is how Team Sacred Heart was formed. I completed five MS Challenge Walks from 2006 to 2010, and completed two Shamrock Half Marathon walks with my walking partner Nancy King.

Adjustments have been made and both Martha and I have embarked on living a healthier lifestyle. When we decided to no longer participate in the MS Challenge Walks, I needed another outlet for my physical activity. She suggested I join the gym which she had recently joined because Curves was closing up soon. I cannot thank her enough, since I really embraced the abundant machines offered at the gym and quickly charted the course to steer this middle-aged body back in shape.

I found it easier to plan my workouts in the morning. So I packed my bag at night and arrive at the gym around 5:15 in the morning. This gave me plenty of time to work out before arriving at my workplace by 7:30 AM. I started out with the treadmills and decided I would start training to run/walk the Shamrock Marathon since I had walked the half marathon several times. In my younger days, I used to really enjoy running. But the older I got, the heavier I became, and running became more difficult and harder on my knees and so I quit running in my early thirties.

I felt myself getting stronger and could run the pace of a mile at an average of 10 minutes. I was up to about 4 - 5 miles before I tore my meniscus which put me out of my ability to run. I decided that my running days were over and there was no going back to that activity. I would have to be content with walking, so, after the surgery, I utilized the elliptical and continued with the rowing machine. When I was at my peak after recovery, I would run on the elliptical for two miles, then row five thousand meters, and then workout with weights for thirty minutes. Around 11 AM at my workplace, I was ready for a nap and often would catch a quick thirty-minute power nap at lunch in my truck.

Martha stopped going to the gym on a regular basis, as she did not know anyone there and it was very crowded. It was unfortunate that her old gym Curves closed. I was a bit disappointed and told her she should go in the morning hours around 9 AM after most people had already come and gone since they would be at work by then. It was just too bustling after 5 PM and she had the most energy in the mornings. She was determined to just continue walks with Sadie at home and doing her yoga. But I knew that was not enough and she needed more of a routine. Both of us had put on some excess weight and it was time to take it off.

The summer of 2010, we began our mission to lose weight and exercise more regularly. We signed up with the program at Tidewater Bariatrics in Chesapeake, Virginia. Their program focused on nutritional education with weekly meetings and you also get to purchase their foods: entrees, shakes, snack bars, etc. The foods were quite tasty and had the proper balance of nutrients. Like any weight loss program, you were required to keep a diary of your food intake, water consumption, and exercise. It is all about counting calories. A fitness program is 80% nutrition and only 20% exercise. It takes the same effort to burn off fat-induced calories as it does for lean-fat calories, so you must eat less and eat the right foods and exercise MORE. We stuck with the program for three months and I lost forty pounds and never felt better. Martha lost twenty pounds and she looked great. I even convinced Kent, my fishing buddy and childhood neighbor, to join the program. He did sign up and he, too, was on the road to healthy eating habits. He lost about thirty pounds.

Chapter 17

THE BATTLES CONTINUE

It does get easier, doesn't it? We would ask ourselves this question often. Living with a chronic disease is no walk in the park. Even though I do not have MS, I like to think that I do "live with it." Seeing my wife affected by the disease and all the twists and turns are challenging at times, to say the least. You give up the favorite "fun" things you did as a couple before life with MS. Yet, I give thanks each day to God that Martha is doing as well as she is. But the fatigue wins more often than not. Martha has learned to pace herself and she usually is able to plan most of her strenuous activities in the morning hours. She has found that if she doesn't rest for most of the morning, she suffers fatigue later in the day.

Once Martha was back on Tysabri, life seemed to be just a bit more manageable and predictable. As she became more confident and positive, I, too, felt more at ease. Together, we had weathered the brunt of the storm early on, and now we had REAL hope for the future. All the information we read and were told by physicians indicated that the present quality of Martha's life could be maintained on this infusion therapy. That was something we could live with. Keeping her out of a wheelchair and a scooter is our goal. Both of us do understand the long-term debilitating effects of this dastardly disease, and realize that nobody is immune from such disability. However, we also put our faith in Tysabri to keep her disability in check and to significantly slow down the progression of the disease. Yet, we also understand her increased risk of contracting PML.

Martha was continuing to speak at Biogen Idec PEPs a few times a year and was even a "big girl" by traveling on her own to give the talks. Typically, they were held during the week, and I was unable to take off from work to accompany her. So she would take a train or a plane and stay overnight. I was proud of her.

Soon, I began to notice Martha's gradual decline in her total energy quotient. The time was 2010—six years after her initial diagnosis. To the outside world, Martha seemed like the same person. But her world at home consisted of more time resting in bed trying to regain her energy. I diverted my activities to do more of what I enjoyed—fishing and playing golf—since she had less energy to spend time with me.

Even though she was relapse-free, Martha continually battled depression and seemed to be in a "funk" and had lost her zest for life. This disturbed me greatly. I tried all approaches to make our life seem more fun; to try and take advantage of free activities like taking the dog to walk on the beach at Willoughby Spit. Nothing I suggested made a difference. I knew I was in trouble. It is the husband's responsibility to ensure his wife is happy, but in this case it was quite a big order, so to speak.

My wife spoke constantly of "hating Norfolk" and "Don't make me die here." We raised our family in Norfolk and I am from Norfolk, but Martha is from Lynchburg. She made the most of Norfolk in her career but still could not find long-lasting happiness in this city.

156

It is difficult to explain completely. I knew when I finished graduate school that I wanted to relocate but did not have any management experience at the time and the kids were in elementary school. Thus, relocation never happened for us. It was not even my original plan to settle down in Norfolk.

When her energy became her chief asset which I had to protect at all costs, I skillfully selected those people and activities that were good for her. I had to be her protector. So, we made the decision in 2011 that we simply could not participate in the MS Challenge Walk anymore. For the five years period from 2006 to 2010, including the MS Walk in 2005, we calculated that Team Sacred Heart raised an amount just over $40,000 for the MS society. We are proud of this accomplishment, but it was not obtained easily. Each year, we had the pressure to grow our donor base, knowing that we could still count on our usual family, friends and core businesses.

With Martha's outgoing personality and the personal connections she had made over the years, it was easy for her to raise funds for our team. The rules of the MS Challenge Walk were that each walker on a team of at least four individuals had to raise a minimum of $1500. The way the fundraising worked on our team, as we grew it, is that when Martha and I had each raised at least $2500 or $3000, we would gladly "assign" some of our monies to a team member who needed it. We added 3 team members to our team in 2010 and continued our fundraising efforts to ensure our team mates would have the minimum dollars required to walk. As we predicted, the next year, Team Sacred Heart was no more. Without our fundraising contributions and planned training walk participation, it just wasn't the same for the rest of the team. Martha was exhausted and just could not motivate herself to fund-raise in that downturn economy.

My job as a Systems Administrator at Langley Hospital was progressing along smoothly. The company I work for had a corporate office in North Charleston, SC. I approached my boss in early 2011, after I had led the site to a successful implementation of our electronic health record system. I no longer felt challenged at work and wanted a more long-term career position with advancement opportunities. So I asked our Program Manager if the company would be able to use me fulltime at the Charleston office and he said, "No problem, we will talk more when it gets closer to it."

Martha and I had decided at that time that we were disillusioned with Norfolk, Virginia where I grew up and lived most of my life. We were fortunate to have raised our girls in a nice house on the river, but now that they were grown and out of the house it was time for us to plan for our future retirement. Our youngest daughter was a rising senior at Virginia Tech. The way I originally planned everything, we would move the summer she graduated since my contract was good at Langley till the fall of 2013.

But Martha seemed more and more restless and depressed, to the point I was really getting worried. She no longer had that "zest" for finding some fun in life amidst the clouds of fighting the MS fatigue on a daily basis. So I boldly asked her point blank, "If I get you out of this house and out of Norfolk and give us a fresh start in Charleston, will you change your attitude, and learn to love 'living' again?"

She gasped, "Oh yes, honey, I promise, if you can get me out of Norfolk. I do not want to remain here and do not want to die here," she said.

So with that, we were both on a mission. I had already realized a few years earlier that our roof needed to be replaced so I had made plans to have it replaced in March 2010. At the same time, we had a bathroom window in the shower upstairs that was just horrible, so we had the same company put in a replacement window in the shower. Little improvements like that make a huge difference.

2011 and early 2012 were extremely difficult times for us and our close friends. We were adjusting to the uncertainty of the long-term effects of this disease on Martha's energy and stamina. Additionally, two of our very dear friends from church died. Tom Pellegrino and our dog Belle both died shortly before Thanksgiving. Then in February, Regina Reeder died. Needless to say, we were both depressed about our situation. We felt we needed a change in order to recharge our batteries.

I noticed that Martha had to rest much more often than even a year ago. If scheduled activities lasted longer than four hours, she would have to rest up prior, and often times I would catch her "taking another pill"— Provigil—to get through the function. Martha constantly pushes herself. But unfortunately, she overdoes it to the point of physical exhaustion, and then she is down for the count the next day. She must remain in the bed and rest until she regains her baseline energy level.

The thing that started to scare me was the fact that I could now visibly see signs of the disease progressing. This progression concerned me like never before.

For many reasons, it was imperative that I "deliver" on my promise to get Martha out of Norfolk and into a positive situation. I too, was ready for our next major adventure.

At this point, both of us realized that staying focused on the end-goal of moving to Charleston, would give Martha enough drive to find the energy to help me get our house sold and coordinate our move. When we decided to make the move, our first task at hand was to get this old house ready for market. We found a show on TV called "Get It Sold." This show was fantastic and gave us some great, inexpensive ideas for fixing up our house. Each day when I came home from work, Martha was so excited to tell me what she had learned and what she had done on this room or that room to make minor improvements. It was re-assuring to see her excited about life again.

The first task in selling a house is to "de-junk." We never had an attic or a garage, so we could not keep a whole lot of junk. I did have a 5x10 storage shed at Uncle Bob's, though. We took each room, starting with my daughters' rooms, and de-junked them. Once upstairs was complete, we tackled downstairs. I made minor improvements to the bathrooms and major improvements to the laundry room. I installed a new drop ceiling, a new subfloor, laminate floor tile and painted the walls and trim. It was a tremendous amount of work. By the time that room was complete, I loathed it since I had labored so much.

Next, it was onto the bathroom upstairs. We figured out how to inexpensively frame the bathroom mirror that spanned the wall over the sink and toilet. I framed it with casing and painted it chocolate brown. Martha had Mr. Johnson spray the shower with a special sealant that made it all one color. Years ago, I had retiled the shower floor with a sand tile. The rest of the shower was 1960's mustard yellow tile. A few case moldings around the shower door opening and the bathroom door, along with new towel racks and toilet paper holder, and that side of the renovation was complete. Mr. Johnson also glazed the porcelain tub downstairs.

I was not prepared to completely renovate my bathrooms and kitchen. The total amount of money I spent on the house, including a new roof and seventeen replacement windows and all the other necessary renovations was already enough! I reluctantly decided to float this on my credit card until closing, since I was confident in receiving a 100% return on my investment in these areas. It was absolutely necessary to perform these renovations in order to sell our house.

I knew I needed to repair the brickwork outside the laundry room at the back of the house as it had separated from the wall at the rear of the house and at the joint on the right side of the stoop as you faced it. The entire laundry room floor had settled over time and this brick wall had moved due to an improper footing years ago. The bottom line is that I knew the situation would not pass home inspection and this would delay our sale and closing on the property.

So I decided to take matters into my own hands after conferring with my real estate agent, who agreed. The thing that really upset me about this entire situation was that twenty something years ago, when I bought this house, the laundry room settlement and wall structure problem existed then. How it passed home inspection back then is beyond my comprehension. No sense in crying over spilled milk, though. In retrospect, I should have made this structural situation an issue when I closed on the house. A word to the wise; make sure you control your own home inspection. Be an informed buyer, ask a lot of questions, take plenty of pictures and document the state of your home at the time of closing.

Once I accepted that this situation was my problem, I had to find a solution. At first, I interviewed several structural engineers who spoke of driving piers thirty feet or so, to anchor the brick wall and drive it back into place. The only problem with that approach was that the initial footing was not deep enough. I did not realize this until I interviewed brick contractors to repair the brickwork on that side of the house.

Affordable Brick Repair was the name of the company and the owner was spot on. He told me, "I used to work for those pier companies and I can tell you first hand that, in this case, it is not going to work since your footing is inadequate." As he was explaining this to me, he was digging around the footing and he revealed its shallowness. He told me at that time that he would recommend demolishing the brick staircase and stoop, and rebuilding it with a wooden one, and then he could remove and repair the brick wall to the new stoop. Finally, somebody was making sense!

And his price was reasonable. All the other engineering companies were extremely expensive, and when I asked them, "So you are going to 'contractually assure me' that the stoop is going to realign with the brick wall when you adjust your piers?"

They all just looked at me kind of puzzled, and then smiled and said, "That is the plan, but there are no guarantees."

At that point, I knew I had a plan and it wasn't with these engineering companies. Even though it pained me to watch the brick stoop and staircase being demolished, it was the correct remedy for the situation.

I interviewed about a half dozen contractors and finally decided on the use of two of them; one to demolish the brick stoop, remove the debris, and repair the brickwork on the back wall to make it a tight seam. The other contractor agreed to build a wooden stoop and stairs. This was an extremely difficult decision for me, as it was not only a beautiful brick staircase and stoop but it also had a railing I had installed years earlier when my children were young, but that railing was not up to code and I knew it.

The end was finally in sight and I held the contractors to a deadline as Martha and I furiously readied the interior of the house for the open house. I planted a few flowers in the front beds and spread some mulch to ensure proper curb appeal. I worked diligently in my yard, to make sure it was inviting. It was the last house on the end of the street.

Selling our house was the first step in moving to Charleston to purchase a new house. We had already made one trip down and another one was planned in December after we were confident our house would sell. We could not put an offer in on a house yet, though, as our house still had no contract on it. Eventually, we reduced the price by nineteen thousand dollars to seal the deal, and we were confident this price reduction would result in a solid offer for our house.

Meanwhile, Martha and I were spending countless hours scouring the internet for our "dream house." All the work was done on our house in Norfolk, and our agent assured us we would get a contract any day now since we lowered our asking price. We had also convinced ourselves that we may have to settle for a house with a master bedroom upstairs as long as it had the master bathroom adjoined, as most new homes do. There just weren't that many one-storey homes or ones with the master bedroom in our price range in Brickyard Plantation.

So the hunt was on! We planned our trip for December 20th in order to find a house. It was a buyer's market with interest rates lower than they had been in decades. We scheduled three houses to look at with our agent as we had narrowed down our "must haves" which had left very few to look at. I eventually had to drop Martha off at the hotel and drive around the surrounding neighborhoods by myself because she was out of energy again and it was a Sunday afternoon and we had to leave early in the morning to return to Norfolk.

It angered me tremendously that she had no more energy for house-hunting. The prospect of returning empty-handed with no prospective houses left me with a burning ache inside. I had to find something. So I drove around for three more hours by myself looking at all our options. By this time, I could now drive by a house and tell from the outside appearance if it had a downstairs master bedroom and what the approximate square footage was, which in our case was anywhere from 2100 to 2500 square feet. Needless to say, I did not discover a house that popped and drew me in.

You need to understand that we only had one house since we were married. We raised our family there, so we were not accustomed to moving from house to house. The memories of our initial house were so vivid and lasting; therefore, it was important for our new house in Charleston to "be the one." It must wow us and we must know from first sight that "this was meant to be." For now, that was not the case. We had to be patient. Knowing this made the drive home longer and we vacillated in and out of depression, anger and hope. In the end, we convinced ourselves that God would bless our adventure and we would find the perfect house.

Several weeks earlier, I learned that my job that was presented over a year ago suddenly lost its funding, but I could not tell Martha because I knew it would send her over the roof! I just prayed that much harder to God that it would all work out. That is what faith is all about. You trust God and put your confidence in HIM. Pray daily and often, and learn not to worry. However difficult it may seem, just take it one step at a time, which was what we did. In the end, it did work out. My future boss explained to me that a decision on the contract would be forthcoming by the end of the month.

Once it was certain that my new job was now in question, my immediate task was to update my résumé and choose a "location" for my résumé's home address. I learned long ago that if you are in the process of relocating, and KNOW you are going to move to a particular city, it is imperative that you make your résumé's home address be the same as your destination city. So that is exactly what I did at this point. We had been looking at a house for sale by owner in Mt. Pleasant and had narrowed down our neighborhood to be Brickyard Plantation.

I had visualized moving to that neighborhood so many times, so I just updated my résumé with that house address as my current address. Then I made sure to go on Monster.com and also update my profile. If you do not ensure those two pieces of vital information are correct, your résumé will continue to be screened for job opportunities in your old home's state. I knew now that my future home was in Charleston. Yes, my family is in Virginia, and I lived there my whole life; however, Charleston was to be my new home. We were setting out on a new adventure which would set us up for the rest of our lives.

At this point in the process, I could not worry about the job; instead, I chose to update the résumé, continued looking for jobs and was even more determined to get a contract on my house and look for that perfect house in Brickyard Plantation. At the back of my mind, I knew that the worst case scenario would be to physically move to Charleston, SC, and still have my job at Langley Air Force Base in Virginia for another eighteen months. I could commute twice a month on weekends.

It was imperative that we find the right house in a great community that met our needs and offered amenities that would welcome visits from family, friends and grandchildren in the future. Such amenities included: a playground, pool, walking, jogging and biking trails, neighborhood boat ramp and boat storage yard, plenty of dogs, and access to the beach within ten minutes. It was totally meant to be. Our real estate agent actually lived there but never told us that until we had closed on our house.

Now that we had a solid contract on our house, I coordinated with my real estate agent to ensure that the appraisal would go through without a hitch and once we had a firm closing date on our house, it was time to find our new home in Brickyard and put a contract in. The housing market was starting to tick up and it was definitely a buyer's market. The mortgage rates were at an all-time low. Our final house hunting trip planned for February 20th, President's Day. There were two available properties for us to look at in Brickyard and we were so excited. We arrived early at 2662 Scarlet Oak Court in Brickyard and the owner came out to greet us. Fred Booth was his name. He asked if we wanted a "pre-tour" before our scheduled showing time and I said "No, we should wait for our realtor."

Martha said, "Sure we do," and followed him inside, leaving me outside feeling stupid. I quickly tagged along as she was chatting away, as usual. He told me that all the lawn and garden equipment and shelving in the garage conveyed with the house, along with a beautiful, red oak and tile inlay kitchen table and chairs that were custom-made. They were moving into a retirement community so they needed to downsize. My biggest concern was also having a fenced-in yard for our dog. He explained that he used to have a dog and had an invisible fence and collar. So that solved that problem. He gave us a brief tour inside. We were so excited. We thanked him and drove around a bit until our real estate agent met us to show us the house.

The most pleasing aspect of this house was the overall floor plan that included a master bedroom downstairs and two bedrooms, a furnished room over the garage (frog) and a full bathroom upstairs. The screened-in porch at the rear of the house was spacious and private. This house had just been placed on the market eleven days ago, so our agent instructed us to put an offer in at a reasonable price. We did so, and the next day, he countered. We had left the hotel to drive back that morning and so we had not received any response since I had no access to e-mail. Our agent finally called us around noon to ask what our response was to the seller's counter-offer. He reviewed the counter-offer with us and told us that we should accept his counter and call it a day. This we did and it sealed the deal! We were due to close on April 20th.

We reflected on our accomplishments on the drive home. "What a wild ride this has been," we told ourselves. Since November, we had listed our house, obtained a contract after a dozen or so showings, made two trips to Mt. Pleasant, and found our dream house and solidified it with a contract. We were mentally exhausted and relieved at this point. Now it was time to kick it into high gear and get the packing underway in preparation for our move.

Chapter 18

THE CLOSING

We decided that we would take some cleaning supplies with us on our drive down to close on the house on April 20th. Moving companies do not let you pack cleaning supplies, etc. So we took them down, our queen-size air mattress, bedding and a dog pillow for Sadie. I had ordered some new stainless steel Cuisinart cookware with my American Express points and had it delivered to the new house. We found a hotel room in North Charleston for two nights and we planned to spend the third night in our new house.

Upon arrival in Mt. Pleasant the day before closing, it was around 3:30 PM and we told ourselves, "We have to drive by our new house and look at it!" On the way there, we noticed a sign at a store on Highway 17 called The Sofa Superstore. It detailed a sign saying, "CLOSING – GOING OUT OF BUSINESS." I told Martha, "Honey, I bet I can get a deal on a chair here." I found the perfect man-chair as I had never owned a recliner before. After negotiations with the sales lady, I received a sweet deal with one minor hitch; my chair was not in stock and would have to be ordered, and the store was closing by the end of the month. I explained to her my situation and said I could pick up the chair during moving week in early May. She quickly checked with her boss and said that would be OK.

On the day of closing, we arrived at the closing attorney's office about an hour early so we had some time to spend. The office was in an office/shopping complex called Queensborough Square and we walked around a bit. We popped into the Publix grocery store for a free cup of coffee and continued our stroll. All of a sudden, I looked to my left and said, "Hey Martha, look over there to your left. There is a chiropractor's office." Her neck was really hurting her and we figured we could get her an appointment later that day after our closing. The practice was called Charleston Neck and Back Pain and the chiropractor was named Dr. Craig Howenstine. We just called him Dr. Craig. He gave us a brief tour, and Martha scheduled an appointment for the next day. She was determined, however, to get a quick treatment from him using his Power Pro Adjuster. That is a device that looks like a big tuning fork and sends pulsed energy through the prongs to treat the trigger points around the neck vertebrae. Martha said it felt great. The device makes a "rat-tat-rat-tat" type of sound. When we checked out at the front desk, Julie, the receptionist, suggested that we purchase the ice gel pack that we could put in a pillow case for twenty minutes on at a time, to relieve Martha's neck pain. It was only $5, so that was a no-brainer.

Closing took way too long. I have never seen so many darn papers in my life. It was a lot simpler twenty-six years ago. Plus, the closing before ours was delayed due to the late arrival of one of the parties. Three hours later, it was done. Now 2662 Scarlet Oak Court was officially ours. We received all the outstanding keys and KEYFOB to the amenities center at closing. We thanked our agent, the owners, and said our goodbyes. After closing, we went back to the bank so I could withdraw cash. We had seen a tent sale for RUGS by the Trader Joe's store off Highway 17 and we had already picked out our three oriental machine-made rugs for purchase. I arrived with $1,000 cash and spoke with the owner who was holding the rugs we had already picked out. He showed me the rugs and said, "The man who first showed you the rugs was my temporary help and he misquoted you the price. The price for these three rugs will be $1250."

I told him, "I am sorry for the misunderstanding, but that is the price he told me, and I have $1000 cash to pay you for them right here and now."

He accepted my offer and delivery was scheduled that afternoon between 5 and 6 PM.

At this point, we were tired and hungry and knew that we had to celebrate with a nice lunch somewhere. We asked around and were told that Sullivan's was a nice inexpensive restaurant on Sullivan's Island. We had wanted to go there as I had made three trips and not yet set foot on a beach in Mount Pleasant. I told Martha, "After lunch, I am taking off my shoes and walking on this beach!"

We had a delightful broiled seafood platter that we split, complete with fresh fish, crab cakes, shrimp, oysters, and scallops. Of course, we had to include two Coronas! Buying a house makes you thirsty! After lunch, as planned, we drove down to 18th station, parked, and walked on the beach. It felt so good to finally sink my toes into the pristine beaches of Mt. Pleasant. Sullivan's Island is where people bring their dogs to run on the beach off leash. You can purchase an annual dog collar that is colored for that season for $35 to let your dog run free during off leash hours. Otherwise, the fines are $1035 which is steep. Tourists with dogs should be forewarned.

It was around 3:30 PM now and Martha was extremely exhausted, as the MS was really kicking in and her neck was still bothering her. All she wanted to do was to lie down. I had planned to blow up the air mattress for tomorrow night since we were going to sleep in the new house. I had the utilities cut over into my name on the day of closing. We arrived at the house and we pushed the button to the garage door opener and drove into our new garage. We entered the house joyfully and I said, "Let's go on the porch and I will set up our chairs and you can relax while I blow up the air mattress. Then you can take a nap while we wait for the rug delivery."

Martha said, "Great, I just need to sit down. We went out on the porch and then I closed the porch door behind me. All of a sudden, I remembered:

"Oh shit! I left my keys on the kitchen counter. I closed the garage door when we came into the house."

So now we were locked out. I was very upset at myself, as we had not been in our new house for more than a few minutes and I already had locked us out. Stupid me! I quickly scoped out the situation and realized that all the windows were locked securely, so getting in through a window was not an option. I called my real estate agent and he reminded me that all house keys were relinquished to me at closing. And to make matters even worse, the extra keys were in the trunk of the car in the garage that was also locked. Ugh!

Thank goodness for smart phones; I used mine to call a locksmith who said he would be there within the hour. Martha and I were relieved but, of course, she had to tease me about the situation. Her neck was killing her. We were both physically exhausted and laid down on the hard porch floor while we waited for the locksmith. As usual, in situations like this, I had to hear several times, "I can't believe that you..."

They made for an even longer wait for the locksmith. Before you knew it though, the locksmith arrived and had our door unlocked in less than a minute. They used this device that resembled a blood pressure cuff and just popped the door open. One hundred and twenty dollars later, we were finally inside our house again. I immediately unlocked the porch door, put the car keys in my pocket and proceeded to drink that well-needed cold beer at this point. I set up the air mattress in our bedroom so that Martha could lie down. So much for my negotiation skills and savings on the rugs we bought— that money just paid the locksmith!

At this point, Martha was starting to second-guess my decision making and began to worry a bit and remarked, "What if the rug people do not show and just take our money?"

I replied, "Honey, I have the receipt and their phone number. They will come good on the delivery. They will be here soon. Please do not worry; just rest until they arrive."

Sure enough, the rug guys arrived right on time at 5 PM and brought the rugs in and helped me set them up in our bedroom, my 'mancave' upstairs, and the family room downstairs. Martha rested some more, and then I turned on the outdoor light and we locked up and headed back to our hotel. She was so tired and I was also beat. We decided to stop at a Wendy's and order takeout to eat back in the room. We also had some snacks from the night before. When we arrived back at our hotel, I put the gel pack in the freezer. After a few hours, the gel pack was frozen enough to do its job so I wrapped it in a hand towel and she applied it to her neck for twenty minutes which made her feel a lot better.

The next morning, she awakened well-rested and her neck did not hurt as bad. We were ready to go to our new house and spend the whole day just becoming acclimated and deciding how we were going to arrange the furniture. We checked out early around 7:30 AM and headed straight to the Home Depot just around the corner. We picked out the paint colors for the whole house, the tile for the porch, ordered the microwave, bought the ceiling fan, and I also purchased two wooden Adirondack chairs that I brought to the house and assembled in the driveway.

We had a great day at the house, meeting the new neighbors, taking walks and just exploring. I went up to the Harris Teeter about a mile from the house and bought some fresh grouper and squash that I cooked up for our dinner in my new cookware. Boy, how I love my new kitchen! I finally had some counter space. After that meal, however, I discovered that the vent fan over the stove was actually not vented outside. This, I would have to fix. I added that item to the list for James. Having a vented range hood was a necessity. James assured me it would be easy to do.

Both Martha and I were emotionally and physically drained and I was deliberating about attending early mass before we departed for Norfolk. Our new church, St. Benedicts, was just down Highway 17 about five miles. I had attended this church when we were on our trip in December when Martha was not feeling well. It is a wonderful church; the parish is very inviting and the singing is spectacular. The cantors have the most beautiful voices I have ever heard. I felt totally at home in this new church. The parish has about 750 families. We decided that we needed to hit the road early so I changed my mind about attending church. We said our prayers and thanked the Lord for our new house and asked him to bless it. The next time we'll be seeing this house, Martha will be moving in for good. I had accepted the fact that I was going to have to commute for a few months and live in Norfolk for the summer. Now that we had our house in Brickyard, all I had left to accomplish was to inform my boss that I was moving and I needed time off to move, and to solidify a new job in Charleston!

I was receiving many calls from recruiters about job opportunities; however, not many of them were in or near Charleston, SC. I knew deep in my heart that the right opportunity would come along. A few months prior, I had spoken with Dr. Thomas Chupp, a navy colleague from Naval Medical Center, Portsmouth, about a job opportunity that would allow me to work from home 50% of the time, and travel the remainder. His company was bidding on a project and he wanted me as the lead Training Manager for all navy sites world-wide. I eventually signed a non-binding letter of intent with his company. Now, at least, I had something in the works to hope and pray for, even though it was not certain since it depended upon a contract award.

A traveling trainer opportunity with a company out of Louisville, KY also presented itself and I went through two interviews and actually had to post a training video on YouTube to be screened for the final face to face interview. I conducted a three-minute dog training video. It was real cute. They told me that they wanted me in Kentucky for the final interview and that, typically, if you get this far, unless you say something really stupid in the interview, you will get the offer on the spot. But then, I would have had to endure a summer-long training program in Louisville, KY. I would not have been able to spend time with Martha and Sadie in beautiful Mt. Pleasant. Being there with my wife after this ordeal was more important to me. I also realized that having a position that required 80% to 100% travel was not going to work with her having MS. She needed me on the home front to take care of her and to be her companion. After diligent prayer and deliberation, I called the recruiter and told him to withdraw my name from consideration. I figured that I would take my chances with the Training Manager position.

I e-mailed my boss and told her I would call her to discuss my vacation request. Once I had the signed letter of intent from the other company, I came clean and let her know that I was exploring opportunities in the Charleston area and that I had bought a house and was moving. I explained to her that I was prepared to commute to Norfolk and work my job at Langley as long as it took. That contract was good until September 2013, so I knew I still had a job. Today, many folks live in one state and work in another, so this was not unusual. She approved my vacation plans and now knew that I was serious about relocating to Charleston. I e-mailed her a copy of the signed letter of intent just to let her know that I was serious about looking for another opportunity but did not want to jeopardize my current position at Langley. It was a tenuous situation and I was not exactly sure how to handle it at first, so I consulted with one of my old bosses whom I deeply respected. She offered me great advice and it worked.

My next project was to interview moving companies since I was paying for my own move. This aspect of moving was quite an education. I received quotes ranging from $4,500 to $8,000, with me doing all the packing. I had budgeted about $5,000 for the move. All in all, I spoke with six moving companies and finally selected Harrison's Moving & Storage after a recommendation from my friend. His price was the lowest, as I made him match it with my other lowest quote. I was confident that I made the best selection. So, to make a long story short, moving day came and it went off without a hitch.

The two most critical points that meant so much to me were the help that each of my sisters provided. My sister Amy who lived in town agreed to send her cleaning lady over to my house once I was completely moved out, and she paid for it. This was such a big relief as I was totally exhausted. Amy also planned a wonderful dinner for us, put us up for the night and cooked us a great send-off breakfast the next morning. We had an entertaining evening telling stories at the dinner table.

The other major stress point that was relieved for me was how to drive Martha down to Charleston in her own vehicle, as I had my trailblazer packed to the hilt with stuff and our dog Sadie in the back. I knew that Martha was not physically capable to drive herself down to Charleston. Weeks before, I worked it out with Elaine, my sister in Richmond, to drive down with Martha. She would stay with us for the weekend and would catch the train back to Richmond on Monday. The movers were not due to arrive until Monday, so we could just have a chill weekend. We had air mattresses so we were set.

Having a relationship again with my sisters was important to me, and that relationship included having Martha want to be around them. For many reasons, there was a falling out between my sisters and me years ago over the family beach house. Relations were strained, to say the least, and I did not speak with them on a regular basis or even see them often. I knew that the events leading up to my move to Charleston facilitated the "healing process" between all of us. I told Martha that both of us needed to "leave the old tapes" we used to play in our head behind us when we left Norfolk. This was a totally new beginning for us. My family was now healed, and everyone was excited for us. Time truly does heal all wounds.

Chapter 19

MOVE-IN

The trip down was pleasant, and Sadie rode in the back of the trailblazer nuzzled in her soft, brown doggie pillow, surrounded by the belongings I needed for the weekend. She was so sweet and I was totally impressed at how calm she was. Dogs know when something big is up and change is in the air. She, too, was excited. We stopped at rest areas about every two hours to stretch our legs and to let Sadie pee.

As we approached the outskirts of North Charleston, I called Martha and Elaine on the phone and expressed my excitement, and I reassured them that we were almost there. Another twenty minutes and we would finally be in our new home. It was a beautiful day and the view at the top of the James Edwards Bridge overlooking the Wando River from I-526 was spectacular. Once we exited onto Long Point Road and traveled down the oak-laden street with Spanish moss, we knew we were finally home. Our journey was nearing completion. In just a few minutes we would be turning into Brickyard Plantation off of Highway 17.

What an absolute pleasure it was to drive up to our new house in Brickyard Plantation. Sadie was so excited to arrive when I let her out of the truck. She ran around the yard a few times, chasing after squirrels. I said a quick prayer of thanks to the Lord for our safe arrival and the beginning of our new adventures in Mt. Pleasant. I continued to unload both cars and Elaine assisted Martha in cleaning the bathrooms. We had to borrow a vacuum cleaner from one of the neighbors as ours was on the moving van. The house was quite dusty from all the painting and drywall work, but it looked beautiful. We were so pleased with our color selections. I popped in on our neighbors who live across the street to borrow their air mattress for Elaine. They are the nicest couple and have a ten years old daughter.

Once we got our beds set up and the house cleaned and got some food in the refrigerator, it was time to go out and eat dinner. Elaine treated us to dinner up at the Break Room. It is the local hangout at the quaint shopping center complex at the entrance to Brickyard. Martha and I had eaten lunch there on our trips down here before and the food was good. We relaxed, met some of our new neighbors and enjoyed our dinner. We knew at that point how much fun it was going to be down here. I told Elaine that we were just going to have some fun while she was here since there was not much unpacking to do because the moving van would not arrive until Monday morning.

The bulk of my Saturday was spent working in the yard, as it needed attention. The lawn mower cranked up easily and I cut the grass and pruned trees and shrubbery. This yard was large enough to challenge me but not too large to overwhelm me. It was just the right size. The wireless invisible fence I ordered was due to arrive on Wednesday. I was able to take the whole week off from work. My goal was to work 10 - 12 hour a day to get us moved in as much as possible since I had to take the train back to Norfolk on Sunday to work out the remainder of my contract at Langley Air Force base in Hampton, Va.

On Sunday, we traversed downtown to the City Market. Elaine had never been there and we wanted to show it to her. The weather was warm so I knew we only had a few good hours until Martha's energy began to drain as usual. MS really does suck from that perspective. I think that the fatigue one gets with MS is the most disheartening aspect of this disease. It just literally sucks the zip out of your step and changes your plans. Any major activities we enjoy are typically in the morning hours. If it falls in the afternoon, Martha must rest most of the day in preparation for it. After we walked around a bit, I treated the girls to Sunday brunch at Fleet Landing. Our neighbors recommended it. The three of us could not pass up the brunch special so we ordered Crab Benedict and it was delightful. The restaurant has seating outdoors on the patio overlooking the harbor and it was a real treat to sit out there and smell the salty air and take in the beauty of Charleston Harbor.

Elaine and I took a nice long walk with Sadie later that day and Martha rested. Our new neighborhood was exhilarating, with the walking trails and cul-de-sac layout. Brickyard was definitely a dog lover's neighborhood. We saw dogs everywhere. Sadie pulled me as usual on the tape leash, in search of squirrels. She made new doggie friends at every turn.

After our walk, Elaine, Martha and I sat out on the porch and reminisced about how nice our trip down here was and the fact that Elaine could be with us. The driver of the moving company finally called me on Sunday afternoon to coordinate delivery on Monday and to give me the final balance for payment which was due. I told him that I had to leave early that morning and would be back around 10:30 AM with a cashier's check and he said there was no problem. He indicated he could start moving in stuff early if I was not there. I cooked us up some grub that night and I continued to piddle around in the garage.

The next morning, I was scheduled to take Elaine to the train station by 9 AM. The movers were due early as well. It was around 7:45 AM and the driver called me on my cell phone as I was in the garage, and I saw the moving van coming down the road. I moved the cars to make room for him. He was really pleasant and asked me to conduct a quick tour to let him know what furniture from the old house went in which room in this house. I had labeled the rooms according to the boxes to make it easier for him. He said, "I got it, thanks."

None of his helpers showed up. He started to move items in by himself and Elaine said goodbye to Martha and I took her to the train station. She and I said goodbye at the *ole* Amtrak station, and she was off to Richmond. I went to the bank to get checks and cash for the movers, tile guy and the painters, respectively. I knew this was going to be about a $9000 week. I always get nervous spending that kind of money but I had planned for this.

When I returned home, the move-in was well underway and it was exciting! First things first; the mover wanted to confirm I had his check so I showed it to him and left it on the counter. His helpers never showed up, so I offered to help him however I could. I reassured him at that point that he was getting tipped for all three of them! I carried in some of the boxes labeled by room and stored them in the closets for the meantime. It was a busy day, to say the least.

James showed up around 11 AM and it was a pleasure to finally meet him. He was very proud of the tile job that Marcos did on the porch floor and he was elated to see our satisfaction with the painting job on the house. I paid James $1500 to give to Marcos for the tile job and $1000 to give to the painters. I would pay the balance of $500 the next day after they came by and did spot painting and painted the garage floor. It was truly amazing what James pushed this crew to accomplish to meet our deadlines. We were extremely pleased.

Over the course of that week, I completed the majority of the move-in chores, facilitated the hookup of direct TV, new phone and internet service and worked on placing the flags for the invisible fence. One of my new neighbors, Brian, told me that I should place the transmitter in the attic, for improved coverage. That is exactly what I did. I expressed to Martha that I needed to experience the shock of the collar if I was going to subject my dog to it. So I held it in my hand at the height of the dog and approached the border and in doing so, it beeped at me and finally shocked me. On the lowest level, it was sort of a tingle so I knew I had to go up a notch. And that notch delivered quite a jolt! I dropped the collar upon being shocked. I felt trepidation about Sadie experiencing such a jolt but knew it would only take one or two jolts in order to train her on the boundaries.

But I did not have enough time to train Sadie on the fence that weekend, so that had to wait until I came back for the Memorial Day weekend. At least, I confirmed the proper setting for the collar and the border marked with the flags. Sadie was happy just to be leashed to the tree in the side yard for the time being. She enjoyed that and had some shade and could still see the activity going on in the cul-de-sac.

On Wednesday, I coordinated with the Sofa Superstore to pick up my man-chair which they had initially "lost" and had to re-order, so I was glad to complete the living room with the placement of my chair directly in front of my TV.

On the way back, I received a call from my new boss informing me that the funding for the new job was approved, and she wanted me to come into the office to discuss it further since I was down in Charleston. I gladly accepted and, now, all things were in the final phases. I would start my new job in Charleston on August 1st. I told Martha, "We can do this. It won't be easy but we can do it. I will come down by train about every three weeks for a long weekend."

Martha was relieved as well to know that the end was now in sight for us. This welcomed news sent me into high gear to work furiously for the rest of the weekend to get the house ready for Martha's sister Jenny, and her mother, Charlotte, to come visit the following Tuesday. They would stay for a week and help Martha finish moving in and get the house set up. And, of course, they would have to explore beautiful Charleston and have some fun!

We went to church that Sunday at our new parish just eight minutes from our house. We truly lifted up our thanks to the Lord for all our blessings in this adventure. We were looking forward to being settled down here and making some new friends at work and at church. I tried to spend the day relaxing a bit with Martha and taking walks with the dog, but I could not help feeling a bit depressed as I did not want to leave and go back to Norfolk. It was so nice down here!

I packed up enough clothes to last me three weeks and hopped on the train to Richmond. My plan was to rent a car but they did not open until 8 AM so I would be a bit delayed in arriving to work on Monday. The train ride was uneventful, and I am glad I brought my blanket and a jacket as the train car was freezing!

My buddy Dean Reeder in Norfolk let me stay at his house in Larchmont for the summer. He needed the company, anyway. Dean was traveling a bit also, so, often, I was there alone in his beautiful house. Those were special times as I was still physically and mentally exhausted from the last six months. Just being able to relax with no duties at all was nice. I only had myself to take care of. I needed this for a few weeks to recharge my batteries.

I had fun searching on eBay for some new golf clubs. My clubs were over 25 years old so it was time to embrace some new technology and start grooving my game again. I found some Taylor Made R7's online for $499. The set included a five iron through sand wedge, a hybrid club, three and five wood and an R460 driver. I thought that was a steal so I had them delivered to Scarlet Oak and let

Martha know to expect them. I had arranged to play golf with my manager during the Memorial Day weekend.

The week just after I moved, my Dad had a seizure and was hospitalized briefly. He has a benign brain tumor that we decided is inoperable, given his age at 87. Mom did not want to burden me with this news while I was gone and moving in, but when I returned home, Dad was in the skilled nursing facility section of their retirement home at Harbors Edge.

I went to see Mom and Dad almost daily for dinner after work. Dad was doing quite well. He was getting stronger day by day. He hoped to return to his apartment soon. His driving days were over for at least six months, however. Mom told me to just drive her car during my commuting stage, as my truck was in Charleston. Thanks Mom; that made a huge difference for me during my stay in Norfolk as I could not have afforded a rental car.

In early June, Dad got sick again and had a terrible cough and he was slow to respond, so Mom took him to the emergency room. Dad was in the ICU for about a week. I will always remember the call I received from Mom on a Wednesday morning around 2:30 AM. She stated calmly but with a slight quiver in her voice that "You need to come to the hospital immediately. Your Dad is in ICU and has developed pneumonia and the doctors think he may not make it. We have some decisions to make."

I hurriedly threw on some clothes and rushed out the door. Luckily, the hospital was only ten minutes away. When I arrived, I saw Mom and my sister Amy. Dad was on a respirator. They told us that we needed to change his Do Not Resuscitate (DNR) status if we did not want him to remain on a respirator.

Neither Mom nor Dad wanted this so we knew that we had to change his status to DNR. A good friend from church at Sacred Heart was Dr. Jonathan Bowers, a pulmonologist. We used to joke and say that if Dr. Bowers came around to see you, it was not a good thing, meaning you were in dire straits; however, he was the best physician around and if anybody could save you, it was him.

So when I saw Dr. Bowers out in the hall and I was by myself, I quickly went up to him, and as a friend, I said, "John, what are my Dad's chances, realistically?"

John said, "Typically with situations like this where he has developed pneumonia, if he does not respond within 24 hours, he could die. He seems strong though and that is good. We will know more tomorrow."

I thanked John and remarked, "I have confidence in you and Dad is strong and Amy's prayers really work." During my conversations with Dr. Bowers, Mom and Amy were out in the hall praying.

It was surreal; standing there holding Dad's hand, looking at him in the hospital bed thinking he was going to die. I was not prepared for him to pass at this time. He was too healthy and this was too sudden. Through the grace of God and Dad's health care providers, the antibiotic and steroid cocktail they dosed him with worked and he responded beautifully and quickly. I spent that next night with him to give Mom a break. She was mentally and physically exhausted after this ordeal.

Dad just recently celebrated his 88th birthday on December 1, 2012 and it was a great day. I know he was glad to be around, as are we. Mom is exceptionally strong and she was a real trooper through the events of last spring and summer. It is difficult to see your parents getting older, as I am witnessing. Mom and Dad have always been so healthy and active. But now, they are getting old and are not so spry any more. I am thankful they are in a wonderful retirement home that meets all their needs. With my sister Amy being local in Norfolk, I felt comfortable making my move to Charleston. They know that I am only a seven-hour train ride away and can get home when I need to.

I remember how fun it was to take bike rides with Dean, Jane and Annette when I was in Norfolk. On Saturday mornings, they would ride twenty miles. I joined them several times and decided that I needed a bike in Charleston also. Dean instructed me to purchase a road hybrid bike as that would be well suited for my needs down there. Martha had her bike that Dean gave her. Martha's bike is basically an adult tricycle.

Her bike is called a PAV 3 and it was a wonderful gift from Dean when we left Norfolk. He initially bought it for his wife Regina. I was going to pay Dean for it, but he gave it to us. It was about $900 in price. That bike has been Martha's Godsend. She is able to ride it, at least, three to four miles daily to get her exercise. Her neurologist was impressed and stated that many of his patients with neurological conditions that affect balance would benefit from riding a bike like this.

Long walks are not an option for Martha anymore as her right foot catches and she loses her balance. Martha called me to let me know of her "episode" when she tried to take a long walk with our neighbor Nicole, her baby and two small dogs. After about a mile and a half, Martha was having difficulty. It was an extremely hot and humid day around 4 o'clock in the afternoon.

All of a sudden, Martha's foot gave out and she fell down. Luckily, she tumbled onto the grass on the right side of the walking trail, rather than the paved walkway. Martha pulled herself up and they started to walk again. Martha and Nicole continued their walk for a while, even though Martha felt unsteady on her feet. This is Martha; she always has to push the envelope. Nicole said, "Do you want to rest a while? Are you OK?"

Martha said, "Just for a few minutes," and they sat in the gazebo and rested for a short time. They were on the trail back towards home and then Nicole witnessed Martha losing her balance and was unable to catch her when she fell again. The MS was kicking in and her body gave out. Other neighbors saw this event and came over to assist her and a nice man in a van offered Martha a ride home. She had some mud and grass stains on her shorts. She explained to him that she had MS and the heat got the best of her.

I know this scared Nicole as well. On the surface, you would never know that Martha has MS by looking at her. Out in public, she does not walk with a limp and she looks fantastic and is just as friendly and vivacious as can be. But when she returns home from outings, she has to rest in bed to recapture her energy. She and I really dislike this fact about MS but you have to accept it, like it or not.

From that point on, Martha ceased taking long walks and rode the bike for her exercise. I showed her a couple of routes winding through the neighborhoods in our complex. She liked those rides and often would leash up little Sadie to run alongside her, and they looked so cute together. Sadie truly is an exquisite English springer spaniel.

This became the exercise dynamic for Martha and the dog when I was not home. When I was home, Sadie and I enjoyed our long walks on the tape leash. That dog is determined to catch a squirrel one day—I just know it. She has come mighty close on several occasions.

I was so proud of Martha during her time alone in Mt. Pleasant without me. She and Sadie would literally hang out in three rooms: the bedroom, kitchen and the man-cave upstairs when she would get on the computer. Holding down the fort solo was difficult, but Martha did it. Without the companionship of little Sadie, she would not have been able to withstand the loneliness for three months. I kidded her often that she "elevated" that dog to a human status during those three months, and there was no turning back now!

It was mid-July and my daughter Sarah and sister Amy planned to visit Martha for the weekend, so I had to change my plans and join them. I decided on this trip that we would caravan back to Norfolk so I would have my truck for my final trip home. When the weekend approached, I was so excited about going home again.

On that Friday, I worked a half day at Langley, drove to Richmond to the train station and handed off Mom's car to Elaine who lives in Richmond. The plan was for her to keep the car for her son, since Dad was unable to drive due to his condition. Elaine had a healthy and bountiful lunch packed for me and we visited briefly before I hopped on the Palmetto train headed for Charleston.

The day train has Wi-Fi so I was able to log a few hours of work on the trip down. I always hung out in the dining car for most of the trip so I could work at a table since Wi-Fi was only available in the dining car.

I met the nicest young lady once I had finished working and it was time for a cocktail. I carried my flask with me so all I needed was some ice to enjoy some Makers Mark bourbon. The young lady was in her twenties and was a Virginia Tech graduate, as noted by her portfolio emblazoned with the VT logo. I remarked that my daughters went there also. It turned out that she was the girlfriend of my oldest daughter's good friend from the VT Rescue Squad. What a small world it is! I found out later, however, that she had a major stroke about three weeks after our encounter. Life is too short, so you better make the most of it each day.

Amy and Sarah met me at the train station and we had a fantastic weekend, although brief. They visited the Citadel and the City Market while I battled the heat and worked in the yard for hours. We enjoyed a tasty meal that evening as I grilled some chicken and we ate on the porch.

Around 9:30 PM, my cell phone rang but I did not hear it. I noticed I had a voice mail message when I awoke around 2:30 AM to take a pee and it was Elizabeth Alexander, Dean's daughter. I listened to the message to discover that my buddy Dean had a mild stroke that morning and he was in the hospital.

On the trip back to Norfolk, my cell phone rang and it was Jane Pellegrino. She informed me that Dean had a mini stroke on Saturday and was in the hospital for a few days. She stated it was mild and he was conscious and alert but had difficulty speaking clearly. I thanked her for giving me an update and let her know that Elizabeth had called me the night before to inform me. I decided that I would drive straight to the hospital upon my return to Norfolk to go visit Dean.

When I arrived at the hospital and was up in Dean's room, it did not take up to five minutes before our priest Father Dan walked in to visit Dean to pray with him and administer the anointing of the sick sacrament, and to give him the Eucharist. We prayed together and it was special. Dean was discharged from the hospital on Tuesday as he was progressing quickly. Arrangements were made for speech therapy. I felt a little bit guilty since I was leaving Norfolk for good in less than two weeks, and Dean needed me more now than ever before. He had good support with Jane and Annette and his family though, so I knew he would be OK. We developed camaraderie during my visit and I appreciated his hospitality and I prayed for him to have a quick and full recovery.

As my time in Norfolk was nearing an end, I had some mixed feelings about leaving. Dad was on the mend but I knew now that he and Mom were entering the next phase of their life. I love them dearly but they are getting old and age is finally catching up with them. Also, I realized that Dean's full recovery would take some time, probably about four months. I reflected often during my commutes to Charleston on the train when I had a lot of time to ponder that truly;

"Life is short and every day is a gift, so it's best to make each moment count. It's the people that really matter; not places or things. Memories of those relationships are what carry you forward."

I was going to miss my family greatly, especially Mom and Dad but we would Skype every so often and I told them I could probably return home for a visit a few times a year. Thursday night was my last night in Norfolk, so I had dinner with my parents and said goodbye, and then I stopped by my sister Amy's house to say goodbye to her and Randy, her husband. They had company so it was a brief visit. I had seen her more recently since I stayed at her house for about three days in July when Dean's family was in town visiting him when he returned from the hospital. I had to give up my "room" at Dean's so they could stay there. I hugged her and thanked her again for everything and told her we would stay in touch and we would work the Skype thing. I headed back to Dean's to finish packing as it was getting late and I had a long day ahead of me the next day.

The way that the various events in life play out is sometimes amazing. I was able to re-kindle relationships with my family, and I was there for Dean, to give him companionship since he was alone, so it all unfolded nicely. I knew deep in my heart that my destiny was in Charleston now so I was well prepared, and I welcomed the new adventures that would unfold for us. Friday morning came and I awoke early and finished packing up the truck, and then I said goodbye to Dean and thanked him for putting me up for the last three months. Off to Langley to work a half day.

Chapter 20

OUR SLICE OF HEAVEN

My last day at Langley was spent "checking out", saying my final goodbyes, and relinquishing my Common Access Card (CAC) card. When it was time to leave, I plugged in my iPod and I was Charleston bound! I stopped at the store on base, filled the truck with gas, purchased a sandwich, drink and some pretzels and on I went.

Driving by myself, I knew I could make the trip in about six hours, forty five minutes, with minimal stopping. I was so excited when I realized that I was finally going to be home in Charleston for good! The commuting had taken its toll on me. I was worn out and ready to go home. All I could think about was hugging and kissing on Martha and Sadie, and now I was finally going to be with them each and everyday. I was so proud of Martha in her coping skills to manage the home front by herself.

Here was a woman who had just moved to a brand new area with a disease in the heat of the summer, and she had met all the neighbors, made new friends, learned various back roads such as Rifle Range Road, and began compiling our list of places to visit and events to attend in beautiful Charleston. Given the level at which Martha operates on a daily basis, sometimes it is difficult to fathom that she really does, in fact, have Multiple Sclerosis.

I had a nice, long weekend planned and did not start my new job until Wednesday—there were no major projects left since we were moved in already—so it was going to be relax time. I knew I would be spending some time getting the yard in shape. I love yard work but I knew it would take a few weeks to become acclimated to the heat. The weather in Charleston is comparable to Norfolk in the summer, but the heat is a bit more intense.

Martha was quite excited when I pulled up into the driveway and opened the garage door. She did not want to fool with parking her car in the garage, so I gladly accepted keeping my truck in the garage. Little Sadie came running out of the garage with her little toy ducky in her mouth. When I petted her head, she peed all over the driveway. I told her that Daddy was finally home for good and kissed her on the head and then gave Martha a big *ole* bear hug and a kiss.

"Finally," I said, "I am here for good now, honey. It is so good to see you! I love you so much."

She had a cold beer waiting for me and we visited out on the screened-in porch and relaxed. She had some barbecue from Mama Browns also waiting for me. It was delicious. We both reflected on our journey and were well pleased with the results. It was going to be so nice to wake up in my new house and be there with my wife, and not have to commute anymore. She deserved some attention after being here alone for three months. I looked forward to taking Sadie for long walks and Martha could join us on her bike.

Often, early in the morning, I would venture out just before dawn to take Sadie for a sunrise stroll. It was so beautiful early in the morning, witnessing nature come alive in our splendid neighborhood. That crazy dog was to the point where when she saw me walk into the closet to put on my walking clothes and I came into the room holding my socks and tennis shoes, she starts going ballistic, getting so excited and biting at my feet and shoes with total doggy exhilaration. It was a hoot!

I told Martha that I wanted to take Sadie to Sullivan's Island early one morning to see the sunrise and swim in the ocean. She agreed, reminding me that walking on the beach was easier for her since the sand supported her feet better and aided her walking. We waited until that Tuesday as Monday was cloudy. I packed the truck early that morning around 6:20 AM and I had coffee, granola bars, water and dog biscuits. I packed our little beach blanket and the captain's chairs, grabbed the newspaper and then we scurried. Once I put the special orange collar on Sadie (to signify that she was registered to run off leash), she knew something was up and jumped up and down. She was used to road trips in the truck, so when she saw me folding down the seats, she knew a new doggie adventure in Charleston awaited her.

It was pretty cool to pull out of our driveway at the crack of dawn when the rest of the neighborhood was still asleep. Away we went to the beach which was only fifteen minutes away. This is living! Martha was ecstatic as we pulled up to the stoplight at the end of Brickyard. We were headed straight through the light onto Hamlin Road which then intersects with Rifle Range Road, her favorite road that took us to Coleman Boulevard.

As we approached the bridge from Mt. Pleasant to Sullivan's Island traversing down Coleman Boulevard to our left, we viewed the rising sun. That splendid orange ball crept up over the marsh view in front of the island. We both remarked, "Oh my God, this is just beautiful. I love Charleston already. I think we are going to be very happy here."

We arrived at 18th station and parked the truck in the spot closest to the beach since we had Martha's handicap parking sticker. We ambled down the wooden walkway to the beach. When we approached the end of the walkway I took Sadie off leash and let her go. She was so happy to run around as she loves the beach. Dogs were already spotting the beach and water with their dedicated owners. Charleston is truly a dog lover's place. And Sullivan's Island caters to dogs with these lenient off leash rules. I set up Martha with the blanket and chairs and we staked out our position on the beach and then we walked south towards the harbor, holding hands and just taking in the simplicity and the tranquility of this beach scene.

We both commented how happy we were now. We finally had the house of our dreams, lived in a dog-friendly neighborhood with boat ramp access, and were only 10 to 15 minutes away from the beach! Life is good. This whole process of re-uniting with my family, closing the Norfolk chapter of our life, and opening the new Charleston book was cathartic. It was our destiny to be here. As we turned around to spot Sadie frolicking in the ocean behind us, we witnessed Charleston at its best; the sun glistening on the ocean and highlighting the beautiful dunes and shoreline at Sullivan's Island. I glanced at Martha and asked her, "Honey, are you finally happy now?

Martha retorted, "Oh yes, dear, I love it and I am in heaven. Thank you for getting us here."

I knew, right then, that the Lord has truly blessed us and we were in for some exciting times in beautiful Charleston, South Carolina!

THE END

APPENDIX A: MS TIMELINE

2/2004	Diagnosed with MS, started Avonex
5/2004	1st Relapse
9/2004	2nd relapse
10/2004	MRI, 7 new lesions
10/24/2004	Consult with Dr. Simnad
1/12/2005	1st Tysabri infusion
2/14/2005	2nd Tysabri Infusion
2/28/2005	Tysabri pulled from market
5/2005	Biogen conference in Boston
3/07/06	FDA Testimony
5/2006	3rd relapse
6/5/2006	Tysabri approved for release in July
8/2006	Begin Tysabri infusions again
9/27/06	Retire from work on disability
12/2006	Social Security disability appeal
3/2007	Social Security disability begins
10/2007	First Social Security disability check
4/16/2007	New York – MS Simulator
9/2007	Patient Advocate Conference
7/2010	Tests positive for JC Virus
Today	Relapse Free, Slow Progression of MS

www.ingramcontent.com/pod-product-compliance
Lightning Source LLC
Chambersburg PA
CBHW071040290526
45795CB00004B/1233